WEIGHT LIFTING

(Original Version, Restored)

by

BOB HOFFMAN

"The world's leading physical director" - Editor in Chief of Strength and Health Magazine

Originally published by Strength & Health Publishing Company, 1939

PUBLISHED BY O'Faolain Patriot L L C, Copyright 2012

info@physicalculturebooks.com

ISBN-13: 978-1470045418

ISBN-10: 1470045419

Published in the United States of America

To Order More Copies Visit: PhysicalCultureBooks.com

FOREWORD

I am a weight lifter. I like weight lifting and weight lifters. Training with and the lifting of weights, which to me was at first a pleasurable form of exercise, an outlet for the competitive instinct all real men possess, a means of keeping fit in the shortest possible time, has become my life's work.

Once it was said, "All that I am and all that I hope to be, I owe to my mother." I revere my mother more with each passing year, as my appreciation grows for the physical normalcy with which she endowed me. I have reached a point in my life where my age is nearly 41, but I feel younger than f did at twenty. I have such pep and energy, such boundless endurance, that life is really a pleasure. No wonder I feel that I owe what I am today to weight lifting. I echo the appreciation of many thousands of men and women who have built their bodies from physical inferiority to perfection, or near perfection, through weight training, who say, "The physical superiority I enjoy to the fullest measure today I owe to weight training."

Weight lifting is something that the busy man can find time to do. It is an exercise for the strongest, and for the frailest man or woman. It can be practiced at any hour of the day, and in any place where there is room enough to stretch out your arms. It builds the most magnificently formed men in the world. It builds great strength, super- health. It produces supermen, men who can star in every well-known sport. Advanced weight lifters enjoy life to its fullest. No aches or pains, no ills. Since I have been a weight lifter, I am a leading candidate for the title, "the world's healthiest man." No headaches, even minor aches and pains, indigestion or any physical inconvenience for many years. Before I learned of weight lifting I experienced a few physical irregularities. So I know that I am not lucky, I know that the much more than average strength I enjoy, the

3

superhealth, is a direct result of an average of one hour a week of training with bar bells and dumbells.

Weight lifting, I believe, is the best form of training for the young ambitious man. It's good for men and women of all ages too. In a few weeks it will cause the immature physique to fill out, to become a mass of powerful, shapely muscles. In a similar period it will bring back the normal youthful figure of the overweight, of the middle aged and bring youthful feeling as well, youthful health, pep and energy.

I am proud that I am a builder of men. I am pleased and proud to have had the opportunity to meet through this great sport the many thousands of personal friends I have throughout the world. This book is respectfully dedicated to those men who already know of weight lifting. It is written with the intention to tell the uninitiated more about "this best form of physical training." It is offered with the hope that it will be a means of showing thousands of others the advantages of this athletic pastime, this form of physical training that every devotee swears by. If this book is the means of helping American weight lifting another notch higher, the means of revolutionizing the lives of more men who need physical training, I'll be very happy. If a man will try weight lifting for a few weeks he will be a weight lifter for the rest of his life. Sample once the glad to be alive feeling weight lifters enjoy and you'll find the hours spent with weight training to be the most valuable hours you have lived.

BOB HOFFMAN

AWARDS FOR WEIGHT LIFTING PROFICIENCY

The A.A.U. (Amateur Athletic Union of the United States) keeps a record of all national records on the five lifts: one hand snatch, one hand clean and jerk, two hands press, two hands snatch and two hands clean and jerk. The majority of A.A.U. districts through the chairman of their weight lifting committee, also list the best lifting records made in their districts. Strength and Health magazine, the official organ for weight lifting in America, will keep records of the best lifts in the five bodyweight classes on the entire fifty lifts. These records will be listed as world- national, district and state.

The five body weight classes will be 132, 14K, 165, 181 and heavyweight. Any lifter tan apply for a medal or certificate for a lift which has been performed before a member of the weight lifting committee in Ills A.A.U. district or before ten reputable, qualified witnesses. The weight lifted and the lifter to be weighed upon the same scale. Any lifter is entitled to a first class certificate for the highest weight listed in his bodyweight class with each particular lift, a second class certificate for the second weight, and a third class certificate for the third weight. These certificates will be mailed upon request and certified report of the lifting for the nominal sum of 15 cents, to cover handling and mailing costs. Gold, silver, or bronze medals may be had for lifting the amounts as specified for the first, second and third class certificates. Fifty cents should be sent to cover handling and mailing costs of medal.

Record attempts must be made at regularly sanctioned A.A.U. lifting meets or Strength and Health Shows or at least before a minimum of ten spectators.

TABLE OF LIFTING AWARDS

	132			148			165			181			Heavyweight		
1. Abdominal raise	70	62	54	76	68	60	82	71	63	88	78	68	94	84	74
2. Pull over	94	84	73	102	91	80	110	100	90	117	106	95	124	119	98
3. Dead lift	400	355	311	430	385	335	460	415	370	490	445	400	520	475	430
4. Stiff leg D. L.	360	320	280	390	350	310	413	373	330	440	405	360	470	430	390
5. Right arm D. L.	295	265	230	320	295	250	345	310	270	365	330	290	385	355	315
6. Left arm D. L.	285	245	215	305	270	235	330	290	255	350	315	285	365	330	295
7. Press on bridge	200	180	160	215	195	175	230	215	185	250	230	210	260	240	220
8. Press with bridge	350	275	200	370	345	220	390	365	230	710	285	260	730	305	280
9. Press on box	190	170	150	205	185	165	220	200	180	235	215	195	245	225	210
10. Hold out front	60	55	50	65	60	55	70	63	56	75	67	59	80	72	64
11. Crucifix	100	90	85	116	100	96	115	105	95	120	110	100	130	120	110
12. Lateral raise	75	67	59	80	72	64	89	75	68	90	88	76	95	85	75
13. Two hands curl	113	103	91	125	112	99	130	120	105	145	130	115	155	140	125
14. Back hand curl	95	85	75	105	95	85	115	100	85	120	105	90	125	110	95
15. Right hand curl	70	62	55	75	67	60	80	72	63	87	78	62	95	85	75
16. Left hand curl	65	57	50	70	62	55	75	67	58	81	72	63	85	78	71
17. Right hand M. P.	65	77	60	90	81	72	95	85	75	108	90	80	105	95	85
18. Left hand M. P.	85	77	60	90	81	77	95	85	75	100	90	80	105	95	85
19. Left hand S. P.	127	109	101	135	112	119	135	127	119	141	133	125	147	137	129
20. Right hand S. P.	132	114	106	131	125	115	140	133	124	146	138	130	152	142	134
21. Deep knee bend	300	275	250	325	300	275	350	325	300	375	350	325	400	375	350
22. Deep knee on toes	140	115	90	155	130	100	165	140	115	170	150	125	190	165	140
23. Rowing motion	140	115	90	155	130	100	170	142	115	185	155	125	200	170	140
24. Leg press	400	350	300	430	385	335	470	420	370	510	455	413	550	490	430
25. Leg biceps curl	70	62	50	75	67	60	80	72	63	87	78	69	93	84	75
26. Half knee bend	450	400	350	490	440	390	530	480	430	565	515	465	600	545	490
27. Straddle lift	450	400	350	490	440	390	530	480	430	565	515	465	600	545	495
28. Leg raise	45	37	30	50	42	35	55	42	40	60	53	45	65	58	50
29. Alternate press	65	78	70	90	88	80	105	98	90	115	108	100	125	118	110
30. Bend over	150	125	100	175	140	115	200	160	130	225	190	155	250	220	190
31. Two hands press	165	145	125	175	155	135	190	170	150	205	180	155	215	195	175
32. Press behind neck	145	130	110	155	138	118	165	150	132	180	160	135	190	172	155
33. Repetition press	130	124	118	146	132	118	160	146	133	172	152	132	180	164	148
34. Two hands snatch	170	153	140	185	170	155	200	185	170	215	200	185	230	215	200
35. Dead hang snatch	145	130	125	160	145	130	195	180	165	210	195	180	225	210	195
36. Repetition snatch	135	140	125	170	155	140	180	170	155	195	180	170	210	195	180
37. Right hand snatch	130	115	105	140	126	115	150	137	125	158	145	126	165	150	135
38. Left hand snatch	120	112	100	135	122	110	145	132	120	150	140	127	160	145	130
39. R. H. clean and jerk	145	130	115	155	140	128	170	155	140	180	165	150	190	175	160
40. L. H. clean and jerk	140	125	115	150	135	120	165	150	135	175	160	145	185	170	153
41. Right hand swing	115	105	95	135	125	115	145	135	120	150	140	122	165	150	135
42. Left hand swing	120	110	100	130	118	105	140	125	110	150	134	120	160	145	130
43. Two hands C. and J.	220	200	180	240	220	200	260	240	220	280	360	240	300	250	250
44. Dead hang clean	210	190	170	230	210	190	255	235	215	275	255	235	290	270	250
45. Continental jerk	230	210	190	250	230	210	275	255	235	290	270	250	310	290	270
46. Jerk behind neck	230	200	180	240	220	200	265	245	225	285	265	245	300	280	260
47. Continental press	175	155	135	190	170	150	205	190	170	215	200	180	230	215	190
48. Bent press right	175	155	135	190	170	150	205	185	165	215	195	175	225	205	185
49. Bent press left	170	150	130	185	165	145	200	180	160	210	190	170	220	200	180
50. Two hands anyhow	210	190	170	225	205	185	240	220	200	260	240	220	280	260	240

CONTENTS

Weight Lifting!

A little-known sport to the general public, understood by few of the sports writers of the daily papers, yet a branch of athletics that is more generally practiced than any other sport or game except running or swimming. In 52 countries of the world, weight lifting is an organized and recognized sport. In a great many other countries there are scattered devotees of this fine athletic pastime to which this book is dedicated.

Weight lifting has been a part of the Olympic games since the inception of the modern games at Athens in 1896. The competitors were entirely European in the early years of Olympic weight lifting. In 1928, the lifting world was startled when El Said Nosseir of Egypt won the world's title in the 181-pound class. In 1932, at the Olympics of Los Angeles, the United States was represented with a full team, and there were scattered lifters from other countries. In 1936 at the Berlin Olympics, 23 countries were represented in the weight lifting. Some of them were Egypt, Germany, Austria, Czechoslovakia, England, France, Italy, Latvia, Sweden. Lithuania. Siam, Malay Peninsula and Argentina. In addition there arc other countries that have record-breaking lifters who are not members of the International Federation of Weight Lifting and do not compete in the Olympics. Notable among these is Russia. At present there are great lifters in China, all the Pacific Islands, India, Fiji, Sumatra, Guam, Cuba, Hawaii, Java, Japan, Philippine Islands, Puerto Rico, Panama, and Colonial British Empire. Armenia, never represented at the Olympics, has a young heavyweight exceeding world's records.

No country, race or color has a monopoly on strong men. They abound in every nation. Only the proper training methods and enough ambition are required for any nation to put forth lifters who compare favorably with the world's best. There are few big men in Oriental countries, but amazingly powerful little men are legion. Just as Japan, through study, application and proper training methods, came up to excel the world in many branches of athletics, champion lifters are being developed in every section of the world. My own pupils are to be found in 42 countries of the globe. They follow the York training system, which has gained increasing renown with each passing year.

Back in the closing years of the last century, there were many thousands of men who set out to build muscles and strength like the great, immortal Eugene Sandow's. So there were lifters in this country in the early years of the 20th century. But the sport went nowhere in particular for quite a number of years. Unfortunately in the beginning of weight lifting in this country, most of the lifters were huge, beefy men of the "Continental" type. They were strong, usually fat, but not fast or athletic. This gave the sporting writers of the newspapers, who to a large degree, mould public opinion, the belief, which they continued to foster through their writings, that weight lifting was responsible for the physical condition of these men.

They were men with huge mastodon-like bones, men who were as ponderous as heavy dray horses. They had tremendous appetites for food and drink and they piled on the pounds. In fact it was believed that the bigger the man, the stronger he would be. Louis Cyr, the French Canadian who won renown as the "strongest man who ever lived," was a typical type. He weighed over three hundred pounds when in his prime as a lifter. Later he scaled four hundred pounds. It was a custom of his to engage in eating contests with other men of gastronomic fame. And he won many free meals in this manner. He and his friend Horace Barre, another strong man of somewhat similar proportions, were well matched in eating ability.

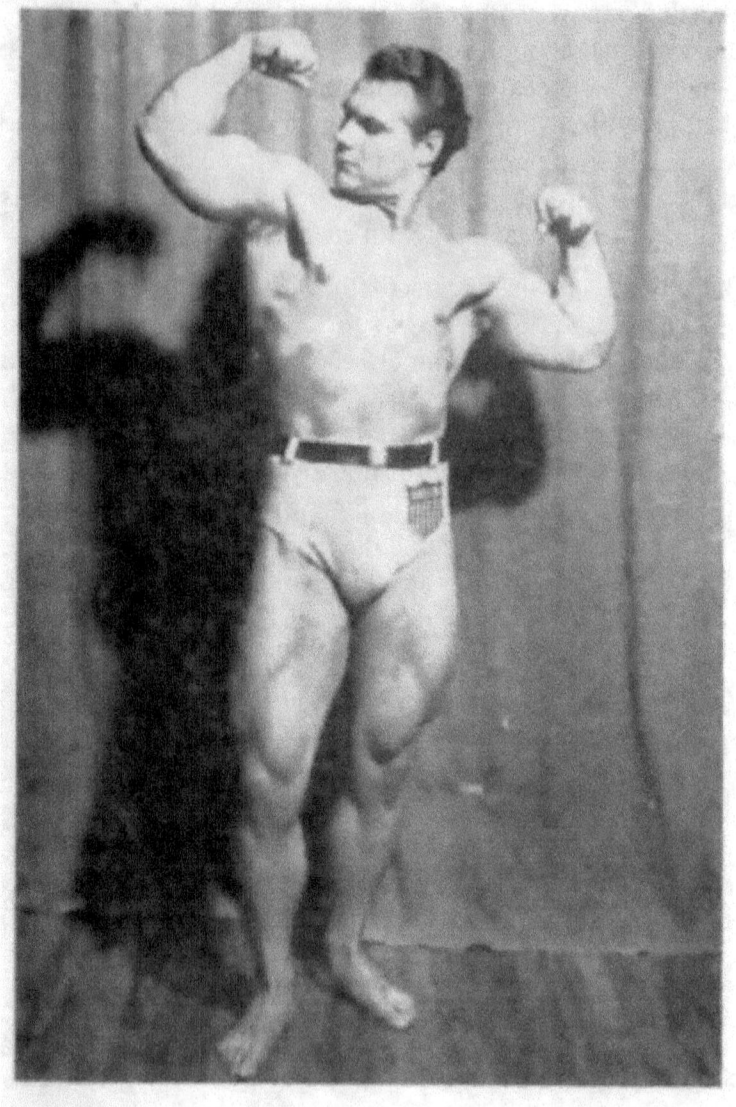

John Grimek, champion weight lifter of North America, 181-pound class.

Only a few of the great European strong men who visited these shores, billed at various times as "the world's strongest man," were normal in development. They were huge, corpulent, slow-moving men. Sandow of course was an exception, as he weighed just beyond 180 pounds, and was an ideal physical type for his height and bony framework. He did the cause of physical training more good than any other one man. Really millions of men throughout the world started to exercise with weights after viewing Sandow or seeing his pictures and reading of his deeds. Of the other strong men who toured this country, Siegmund Breitbart and the Saxon trio are among the few who could be numbered among the really well-built, normal type of men. Breitbart was the last of the great professional strong men to startle the audiences of this country. Week after week, his act commanded $7,000 in the coin of the realm at the New York Hippodrome.

Two of the Saxons, Curt and Herman, were average in size and beautifully built. While Arthur, whom many believe to be the strongest man of all time, was not a huge man as weight lifters went—seldom more than 200 pounds —he had renown as an eating and drinking champion. It was not unusual for him to drink a hundred bottles of beer in a day; so we are told. And every day in his act, among other great feats of strength, he would lift overhead in the bent press style over three hundred pounds. His official record is 371! Arthur did not care for muscles or posing— the direct opposite to Sandow, who is best remembered and most famous for his matchless physique. There are many who believe that Sandow was the strongest man of his time. He was good, but at least threescore of men since his time have exceeded his best records. Arthur Saxon was super- strong; many of his records have not even been approached. But he did not care about his appearance, and did not create as good an impression as he could have done with a little specialization in body building and improved posture.

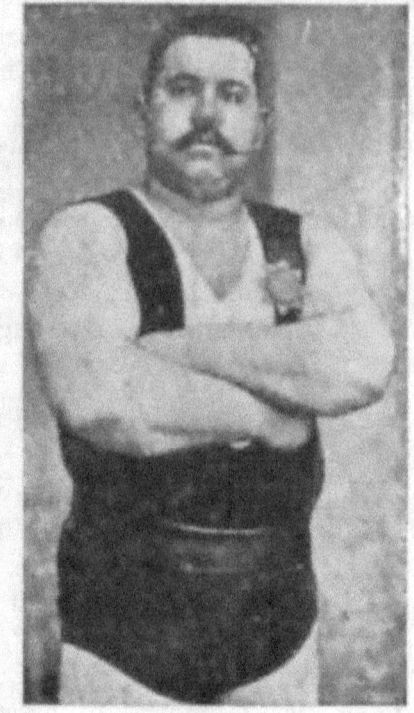

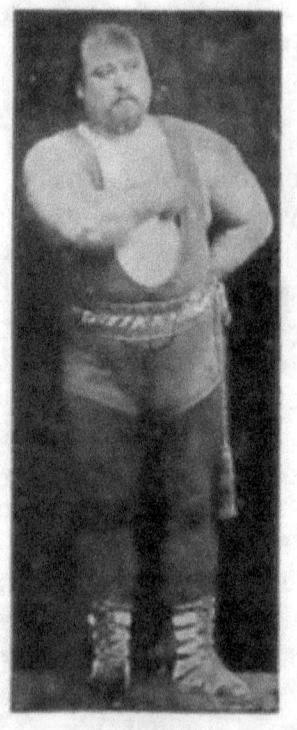

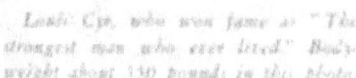

We have already mentioned Louis Cvr and Horace Barre. Then there was Carl Moerke, a man of only five feet four inches in height, 250 pounds in weight, who was very strong, but built surprisingly similar to the farm animal most of 11s know well. There were the amazing Sampson,

Cyclops, Swoboda, Appolon and many others who were very much on the heavy side, and continued the impression received by so many that weight lifting made them that way.

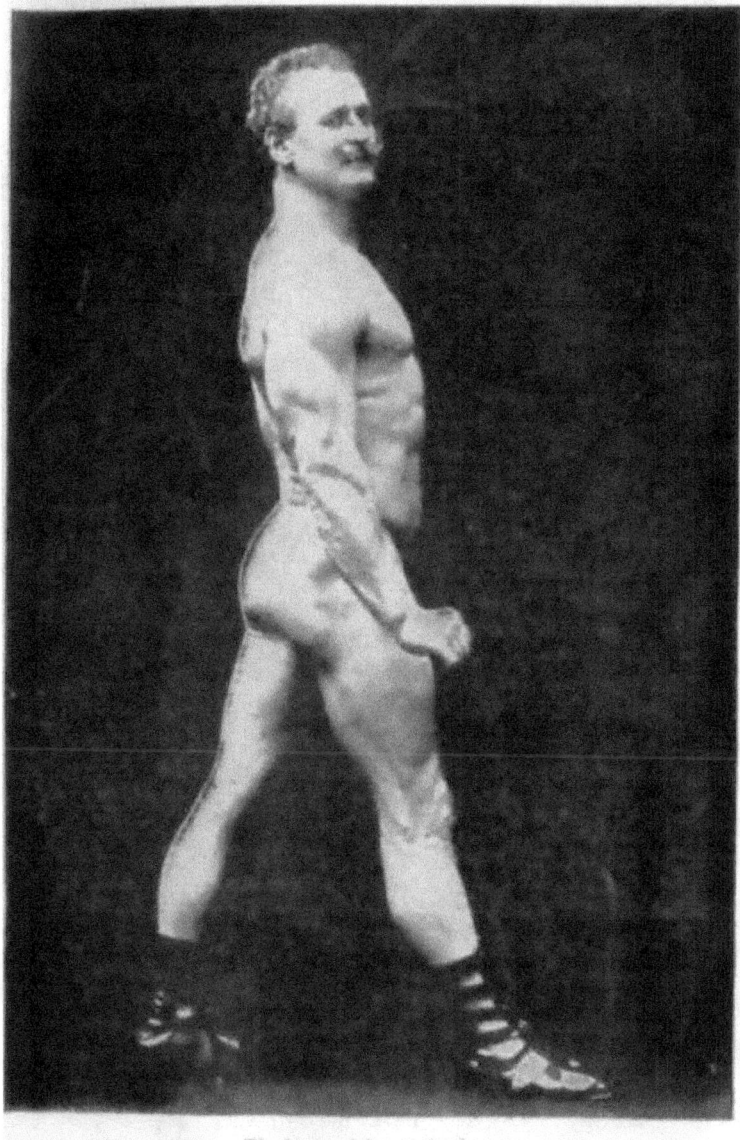

The Immortal Eugene Sandow.

So our favorite game has been much maligned. There are those today who believe that weight lifting will produce lethargic, ponderous, fat men. Those who do not know, believe that it is a slow, uninteresting sport. Yet to many-thousands who have tried lifting, it is as interesting as a boxing or wrestling match. The championships are well attended, it not being unusual for the paid attendance to run into the thousands. If you had the opportunity to walk into the arena where the Olympic weight lifting championships were being contested, you would be astonished to hear the tremendous enthusiasm which is rampant at those affairs. All one need do is to know weight lifting to like it and to obtain pleasure from seeing the best lifters in action.

Much of the false impression concerning weight lifting has come about through the advertisements of the "Train You by Mail" professors, who find it more profitable to sell a course of exercises without apparatus—to sell a typewritten course of exercises for twenty-five or thirty-five dollars. It is expensive to produce well-balanced, well- constructed weight lifting sets. The sets of weights used in actual competition are made with chrome vanadium bars, balanced, machined, tooled to proper weight. And a variety of plates range in size from 1¼, 2½, 5, 10, 20, 25 and on up to 45 pounds or more with the various sets. There is the cost of the material, the labor, the machine work, the painting and packing, all of which makes it impossible to sell weights profitably through the mail or advertisements in other magazines. One of the leading advertisers in the physical culture world today, who built his own once magnificent body chiefly with bar bells, now "knocks" weights and weight lifting in every piece of advertisement he sends out. His excuse as offered to me personally was, "I find it hard enough to sell my course and if I don't knock weight lifting, I can't sell my course at all."

Therefore the world's best form of exercise has been unfairly maligned, stigmatized as a sport which will ruin its devotees physically, building fat, ugly, misshapen bodies, with weak hearts, hardened arteries. These are only some of the things those who don't know weight lifting and its splendid effects upon the human body have to say about it. It has even been claimed that weight lifting makes men weak sexually, while directly the opposite is true, as weight lifters arc the most virile of men. Anything to sell one or two more of the advertised courses offered without apparatus or weights.

Through all of this unfavorable writing, weight lifting not only survived but has grown by leaps and bounds. Like the rolling snowball, it gains greater momentum and greater numbers of enthusiastic followers each year. These arc the men who in most cases tried the other forms of physical training with little or no results. They retained an open mind, heard of weight lifting, investigated, saw some of the amazing physical specimens (many of whom are shown in this book), which weight lifting produced, and they in turn became weight lifters—men who constantly strive to encourage others to enjoy this wholesome pastime which builds so much in the way of strength and health, while adding to the interest and pleasure of life.

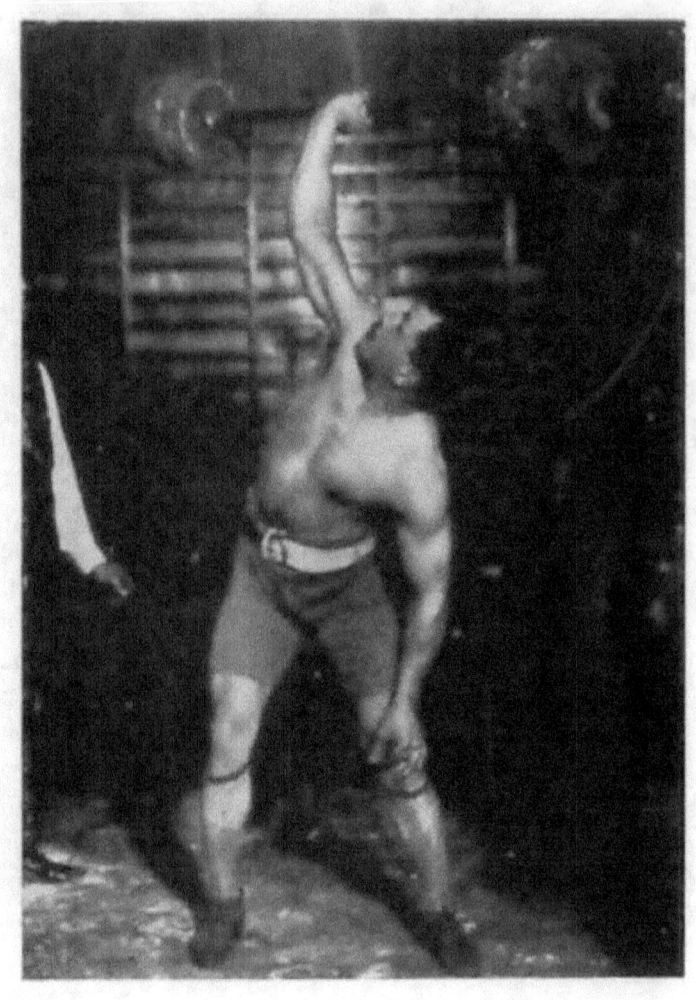

ARTHUR SAXON

One of the strongest men of all time. He holds the world's record in the two hands anyhow lift, 448 pounds, and the greatest bent press on record—371 pounds.

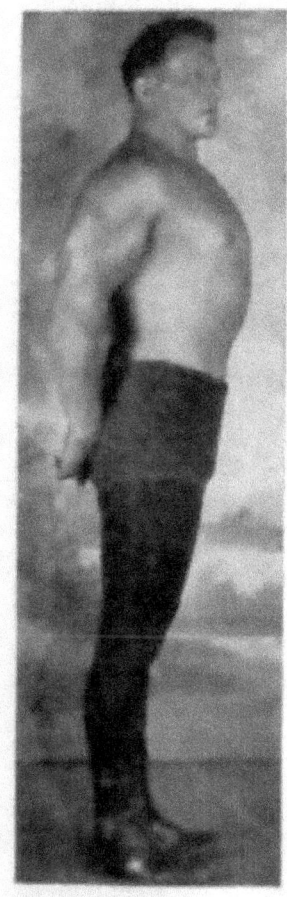

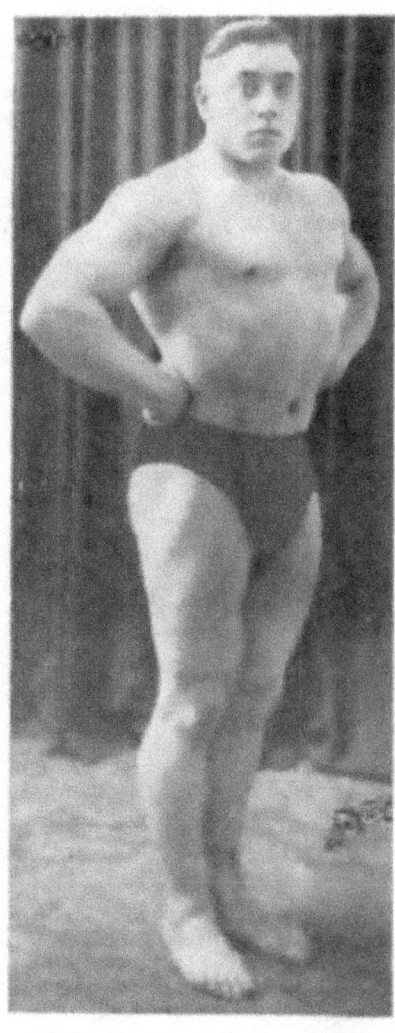

Below — Henry Steinborn,
world's champion lifter of
1920.

Charles Rigoulot of France, who holds
the world's professional records in the one
hand snatch, two hands snatch and the
two hands clean and jerk—264, 314, 402
respectively.

Weight lifting in this country went along for years making
little or no permanent progress until after the great war. By
that time, weight lifting had become an important part of
the Olympic games program. Three lifts known as the

17

Olympic lifts had been selected. For a time there were five lifts—the one hand snatch, the one hand jerk, the two hands press, the two hands snatch and the two hands clean and jerk. Although the first two lifts are worthy strength tests, exercises which will produce so much in the way of strength, owing to the great length of a five lift program, only the three Olympic lifts are now generally the basis for competition in championship lifting.

Weight Lifting in America

During the Sandow era, in America as in the rest of the world, thousands of youths decided to emulate him and become the "world's best-built man" or the "world's strongest man." Only a few of these men are known to the bar bell men of today.

An occasional demonstration of lifting was offered in the early years of this century, but progress in the sport of weight lifting was deplorably slow. On the second day of May, 1916, Joe Nordquest, one of the greatest of native-American strong men, established a world's amateur record of 277pounds in a one hand lift overhead, bent press style. In a sworn statement before a notary public signed by witnesses are a number of names known to the older lifting enthusiasts of today Otis Lambert, Charles McMahon, George Zottman, Teddy Mack, O. R. Coulter, Alan Calvert, Anton Matysek, R. I. Smith, John Lambert, Robert B. Snyder, Jr., and Adolph Nordquest.

These men were the real pioneers of American weight lifting, the men who were establishing records before the great war. They were the inspiration to the leaders of the weight lifting movement throughout the country today. To these early American weight lifters we owe a great debt.

During the war there was little activity in weight lifting. The old Strength magazine was not published during that time and nothing has been heard of official lifting during that period. But right after the war, American lifting received a good push forward by the visit to this country of Henry Steinborn. Henry has been active in the strength world as one of the best professional wrestlers during these many years. But back in 1920 he was a young German, recently released from a war prison camp in Australia. It was there that he had developed his Herculean powers which enabled him to exceed world's records in the "quick lifts."

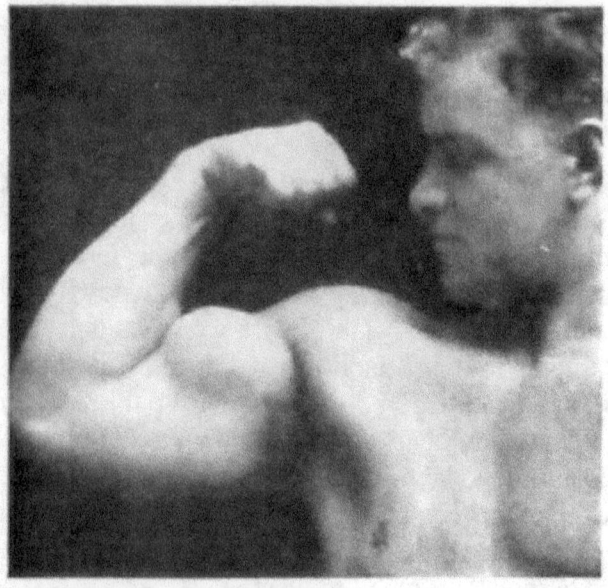

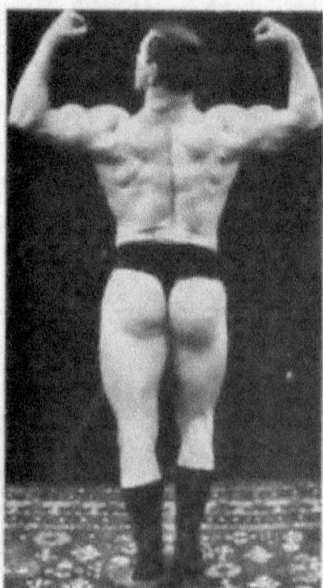

Above—Joe Nordquest, one of the greatest of native American strong men. He made an official record of 272½ pounds in the bent press—388 pounds in the press on floor with bridge.

George Hackenschmidt, world's champion wrestler and lifter of 1908. Now 60 years of age he is an amazing physical specimen who spends his years lecturing and studying philosophy.

Prior to the advent of Henry Steinborn, the lifts commonly practiced in America were the bent press, dead weight lift, curls and two hand presses of one sort and another. But Henry really showed the possibilities of the quick lifts which had become popular in Europe a few- years before his visit here. The one hand snatch, the two hands snatch and the two hands clean and jerk were Steinborn's specialties.

The lifting enthusiasts of the early 1920's' saw undreamed-of poundages hoisted to arm's length by this powerful young German. He exceeded the world's record in the one hand snatch with a lift of 218. He made a two hands snatch of 230 pounds, and a two hands official clean and jerk of 350 pounds, to exceed the official world's clean and jerk record of 347 pounds credited to the great Louis Cyr, the French Canadian.

From 1920 on, there was more interest in America in the lifts which were known as the International lifts—one hand snatch, one hand clean and jerk, two hands military press, two hands snatch, and twp hands clean and jerk. But it was not until a number of years later that these lifts were made the official championship group. For in 1923, the year in which I first learned of and became enthusiastic about weight lifting, the official lifts for the year were one hand clean and jerk, one hand bent press, two hands snatch, two hands clean and jerk and dead weight lift.

These were the lifts that we used in a contest in York which I believe was the first official contest held in America. I conducted the meet, tried to supervise the officiating in seven body weight classes as well as competed myself. We did not know how to properly conduct a meet in those days such its is done today, with all the contestants taking their turn at one bar bell, making their lifts when the weight reaches a poundage suitable to them. I had made arrangements for seven platforms and seven bar bells.

Gathering these sets of weights and arranging the seats and the seven platforms did not leave much energy for my own lifting, but I managed to win this first contest by a small margin.

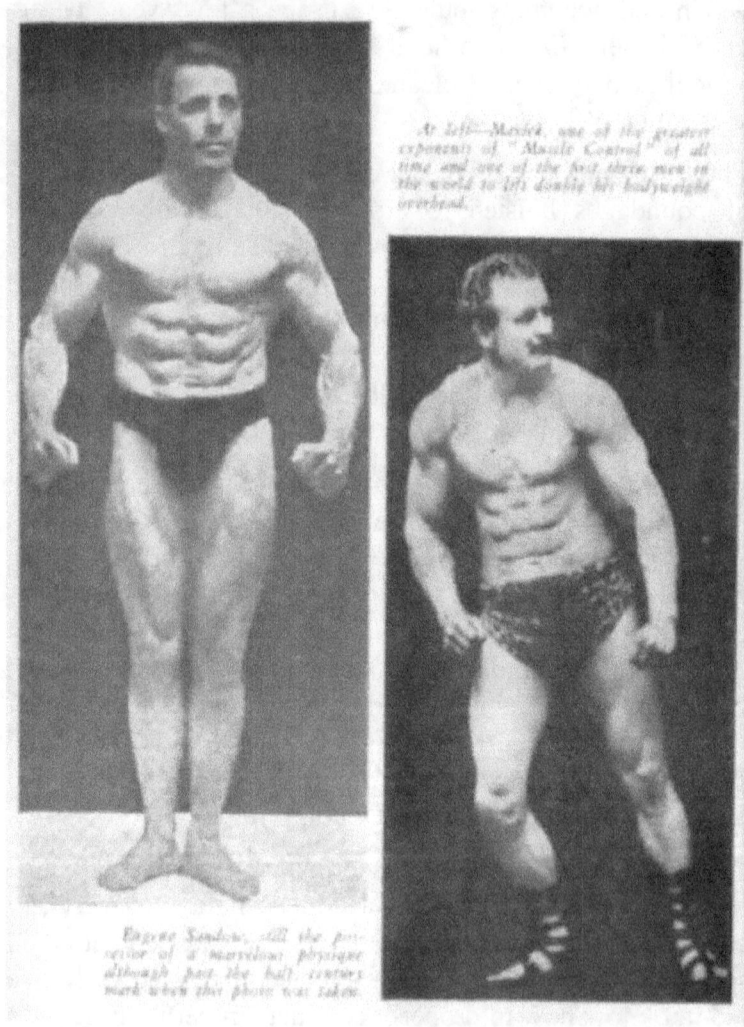

At left—Maxick, one of the greatest exponents of "Muscle Control" of all time and one of the first three men in the world to lift double his bodyweight overhead.

Eugene Sandow, still the possessor of a marvelous physique although past the half century mark when this photo was taken.

Exhibitions of lifting, both amateur and professional, regularly took place in New York and Philadelphia. The usual system was for any man, who felt that he could approach or break a record on any lift or strength feat, to take part in the program. In 1925 certain men" were considered to be "the national champions in the series of lifts for that year. In 1926 at the Sesquicentennial in Philadelphia a weight lifting championship was held. Art Levan, one of the older members of the York team, and myself engaged in that contest. Dirk Bacluell was present and there the ambition which carried him later to nine national weight lifting titles, many records, a berth on the Olympic and world's champion teams, was born.

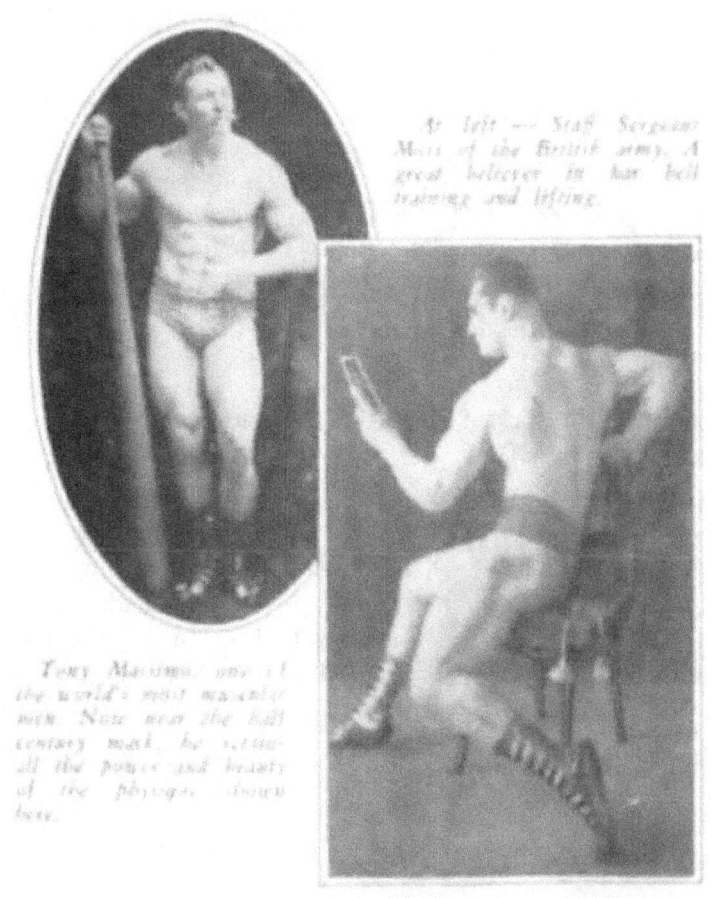

At left — Staff Sergeant Moss of the British army. A great believer in bar bell training and lifting.

Tony Massimo, one of the world's most muscular men. Now near the half century mark, he retains all the power and beauty of the physique shown here.

More than a 200-pound clean and jerk was considered phenomenal in those clays. When I engaged in a contest or exhibition with Al Manger, who was destined to be official heavyweight champion and a member of the 1932 Olympic team, a high lift of 250 pounds in the clean and jerk was the marvel of the American lifting world. During the year of 1926 I fulfilled a long-cherished ambition to row for a world-famous Philadelphia rowing club as a member of their championship eight. This did not permit time for weight training, as our coach, who coached several Olympic teams during those years, was a real slave driver, and an oarsman had nothing left for any other form of training when through with his rowing on the river.

My interest in weight lifting not only continued but increased during this period, witnessed by my stealing away from practice one day to take part in the lifting at the Sesquicentennial. In 1927 there was an attempt to conduct a truly representative, national weight lifting championship. But lifters were few enough. 1 won the national heavyweight title that year with lifts that the best featherweights can perform today.

1929 was to see an important step forward in American weight lifting. That year, chiefly through the efforts of Siegmund Klein, Dietrich Wortmann—still our national A.A.U. weight lifting chairman, then the president of the German-American Athletic Club—became sufficiently interested to approach the A.A.U. and persuade them to take over weight lifting and conduct it as one of the official sports under their sanction and direction.

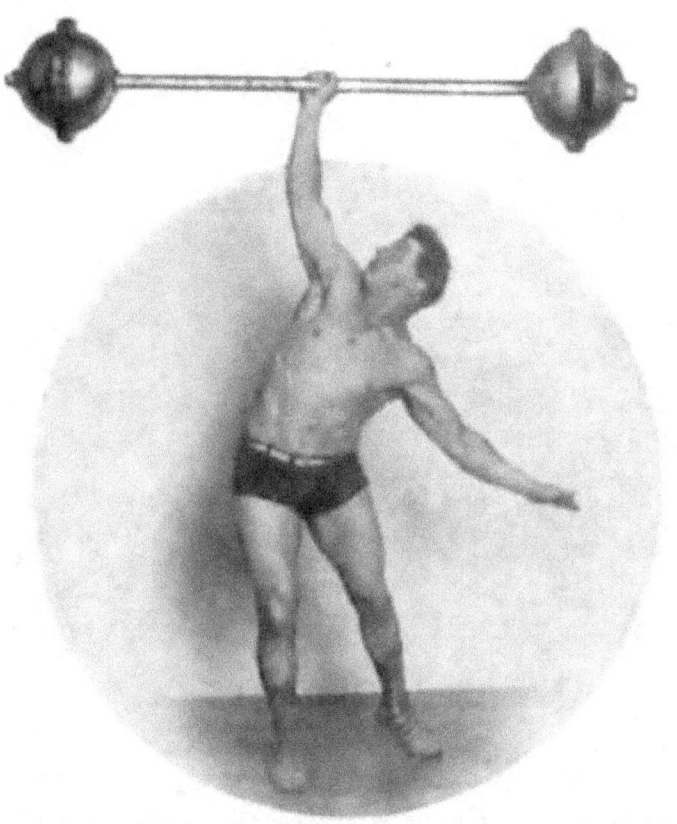

Henry Steinborn at the time he set a new world's record in the one hand snatch and the two hands clean and jerk.

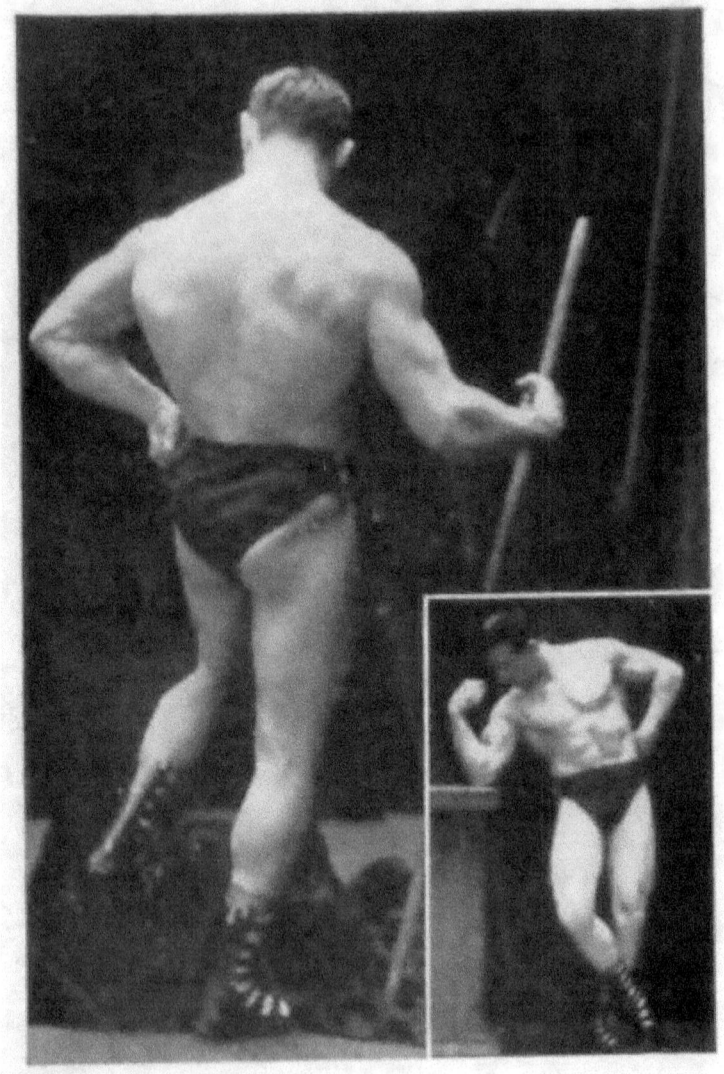

Siegmund Klein, who has won honors for his physique, for his great strength. He's famed as one of the world leaders in bar bell training and weight lifting and will be one of the immortals of tomorrow.

Thus weight lifting became an official Amateur Athletic Union sport in America. The A.A.U. is affiliated with the International Federation of Weight Lifting to which the majority of countries throughout the world where weight lifting is an established sport, belong. So America was ready to start up the ladder to world weight lifting fame.

The first official weight lifting A.A.U. championships were conducted in 1929 at the old German-American Athletic Club in New York. The majority of contestants were members of die various German-American clubs in New York City. Many of the men who entered had had previous lifting experience in the old country before making their home in New York and there were some good lifters present. The greatest lift of the day was performed by Willie Rhorer.

NATIONAL CHAMPIONS OF 1929

	1 H. Snatch	1 H. C. & J.	2 H. M. P.	2 H. Snatch	2 H. C. & J.	Total
118-POUND CLASS Knodle	104½	126½	143	132	176	682
128-POUND CLASS Gaukler	110	126½	137½	121	165	665
136-POUND CLASS Bachtell	143	159½	154	165	225	852½
148-POUND CLASS M. Rohrer	154	176	148½	170½	242	891
165-POUND CLASS Fass	143	176	176	176	231	902
181-POUND CLASS Manger	143	159½	198	192½	264	957
HEAVYWEIGHT CLASS W. Rohrer	170½	198	187	203½	286	1045

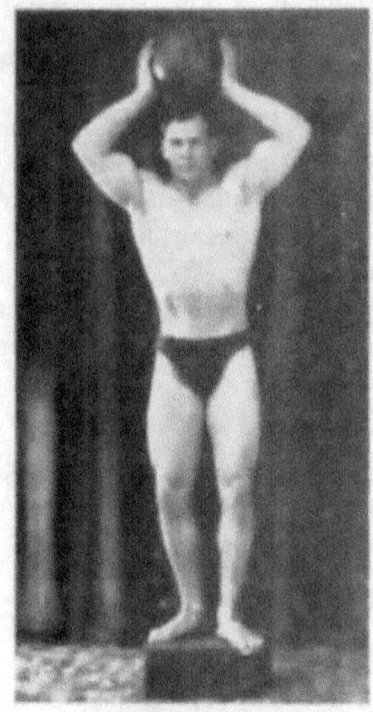

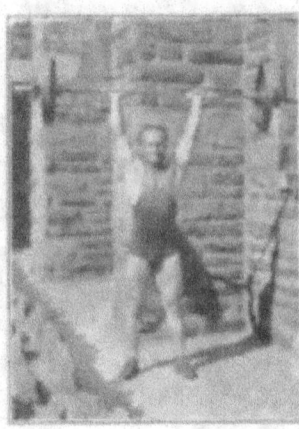

Three famous champions who made their start in the beginning of official United States weight lifting. Above—Art Levan, eleven times a national champion. Below —Dick Bachtell, whose score is ten national championships. Arnie Sundberg, with ball overhead, the champion of 1928, 1929, 1930, 1931, 1932.

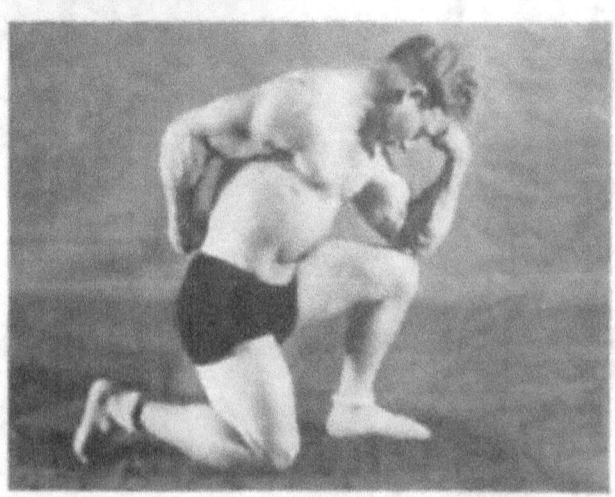

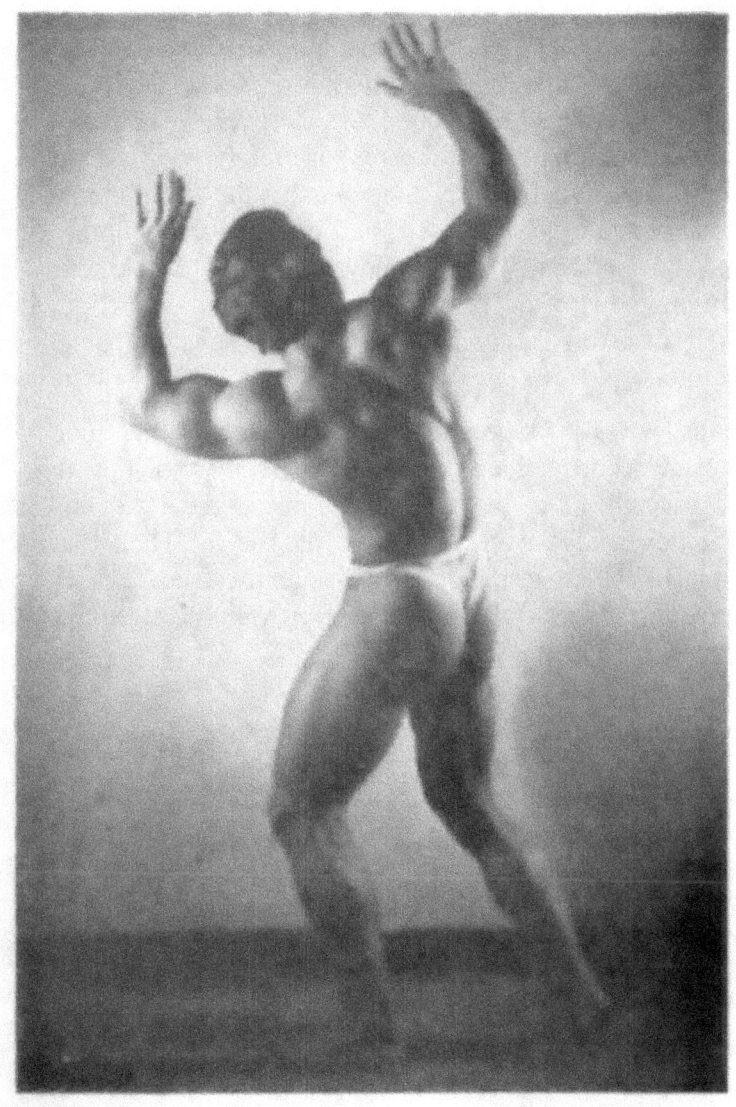

A splendid back pose of John Grimek.

Competitors who were outclassed in this first A.A.U. official contest went home with greater enthusiasm than ever. They trained hard and faithfully during the ensuing year and reported for the second A.A.U. championship, conducted by Dietrich Wortmann's German-American Athletic Club, again in 1930, at their athletic field on Long Island, just across the river from New York. That was a memorable day. I remember it as if it were yesterday. Held in the open, under the blazing sun, really good poundages were lifted. The native Americans for the first time gave a great account of themselves and provided real competition for the German-American boys. I say native Americans, although many of them were of German extraction, but their ancestors had come to this country several generations before.

Tony Terlazzo, at present three times world's champion and world's record holder, considered by many to be the world's best weight lifter, made his appearance first at that contest. Art Levan also won a national title, as did Dick Bachtell and Bill Good in the light-heavyweight class. These men were later to lead the York Bar Bell weight lifting team to the national team title.

NATIONAL CHAMPIONS OF 1930

	1 H. Snatch	1 H. C. & J.	2 H. M. P.	2 H. Snatch	2 H. C. & J.	Total
118-Pound Class						
Knodle	110	137½	148½	132	187	715
128-Pound Class						
Levan	137½	137½	148½	170½	225½	819½
136-Pound Class						
Bachtell	143	165	154	165	220	847
148-Pound Class						
Rohrer	154	192½	159½	176	253	935
165-Pound Class						
Sundberg	159½	176	165	198	269½	968
181-Pound Class						
B. Good	159½	176	203½	203½	275	1017½
Heavyweight Class						
Manger	148½	176	209	192½	275	1001

In 31 the senior national A.A.U. championships were held in Philadelphia at the Penn A. C. There were many more contestants than ever before. They were more truly representative of our nation and the records started to go up. But American weight lifting had a long way to go. For that year, with all the competitors present, there was just one who two hand snatched over 200 pounds. Arnie Sundberg, that year lightweight champion, who had made his annual trip across the country from the Multnomah Athletic Club in Portland, Ore., made a good try with 203½ pounds. But Bill Good's 209 was the highest snatch of the day.

Now hundreds of American lifters snatch over 200 pounds. Terry holds the world's 132-pound class record at 215 pounds. Terlazzo officially snatched 242 to equal the world's record in the 148-pound class. Johnny Terpak snatched 260 pounds weighing but 160. John Davis, lifting in the 181-pound class, made 267 'A pounds, and big Steve Stanko, heavyweight, has forced the national record up and up and has succeeded with 290 pounds. He has had 300 pounds to straight arms, a poundage which would have exceeded the world's heavyweight record, the greatest amateur lift of all time.

NATIONAL CHAMPIONS OF 1931

	1 H. Snatch	1 H. C. & J.	2 H. M. P.	2 H. Snatch	2 H. C. & J.	Total
118-POUND CLASS						
Knodle	110	132	148½	137½	187	715
126-POUND CLASS						
Levan	137½	148½	159½	176	231	852½
132-POUND CLASS						
Bartlett	154	170½	154	199½	214½	852½
148-POUND CLASS						
Horn	148½	165	187	192½	242	935
165-POUND CLASS						
Sundberg	165	176	154	187	258½	940½
181-POUND CLASS						
Wm. Good	165	198	198	209	286	1056
HEAVYWEIGHT CLASS						
Manger	154	181½	198	192½	269½	995½

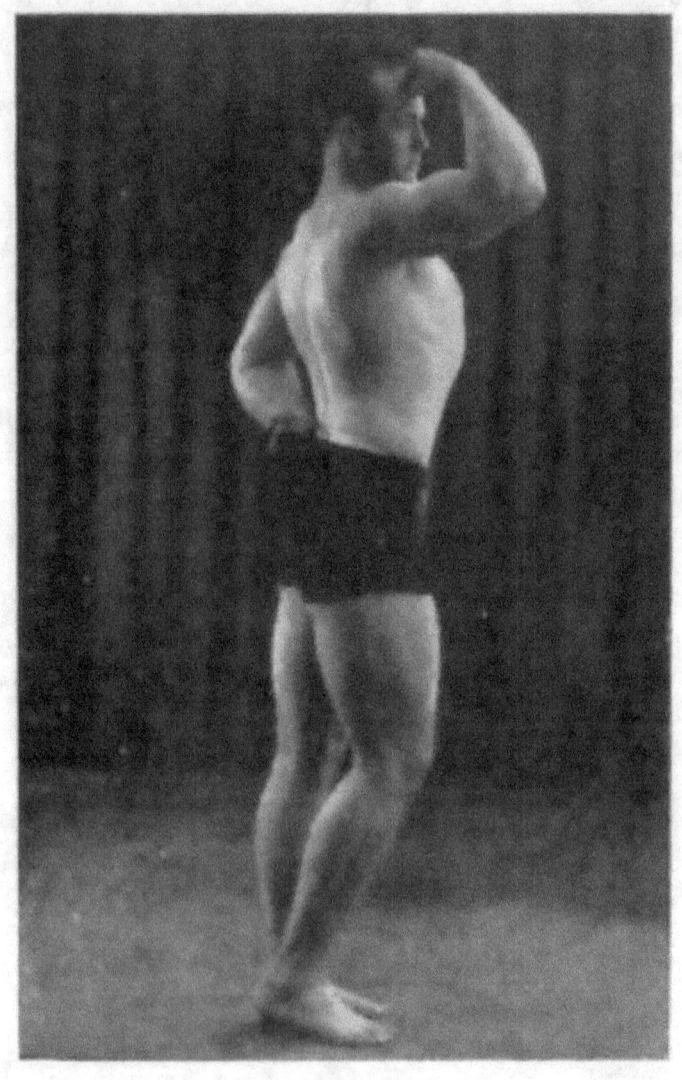

Bob Hoffman, the world's leading physical director. For years Bob has been the world's leader in weight lifting, and is responsible for much of the rise of American weight lifting from its former position of mediocrity to the point where we now have the world's strongest weight lifting team.

The York team, as we will relate in another chapter, was making lifting history, so it was thought fitting that we should he given the opportunity to conduct the national A.A.U. championships of 1932. They were contested that year in the York Y. M. C. A. There were a great many entries from all sections of the country and the contest dragged along from 2 o'clock in the afternoon until after 11 o'clock at night. This was the last year in which there was an endeavor to conduct all the championships in a day.

The York team was represented in all of the classes and won the national weight lifting team title that year for the first time, an honor which they have held from that day to the present. The champions were: Lucien LaPlante of Gardner, Mass., in the 112-pound class; Joe Fiorito of York in the 118; Art Levan of York in the 126; Tony Terlazzo and Dick Bachtcll, both members of the York team for these last years, tied for first in the 132; Arnie Sundberg of Portland, Ore., won first place in the 148; Stanley Kratkowski, who has represented the Michigan Alkali Club of Wyandotte, Mich., for some years, won his first title in the 165-pound class, narrowly defeating Wally Zagurski and Joe Miller of York; Bill Good of the York team won the light-heavyweight title and Al Manger of Baltimore, the heavyweight championship. The champions of 1932 and their lifting totals follow:

112-POUND CLASS
Lucien LaPlante, West End A. C., Gardner, Mass............... 470

118-POUND CLASS
Joe Fiorito, York, Pa. 485

126-POUND CLASS
Art Levan, York, Pa. 540

132-POUND CLASS
Dick Bachtell and Tony Terlazzo, York, Pa., tied with........ 570

148-POUND CLASS
Arnie Sundberg, Portland, Ore. 632

165-POUND CLASS
Stanley Kratkowski and Joe Miller tied with................ 680

181-POUND CLASS
Bill Good, York, Pa. 715

HEAVYWEIGHT CLASS
Al Manger, Baltimore, Md. 704

In 1933 the national championships were held in conjunction with the Chicago World's Fair. Sixty men competed and all the body weight classes were well represented. That year the York team won five of the championships, narrowly missing in the 132 through an injury to Dick Bachtell and in the heavyweight where Joe Miller did not begin to reach his practice poundages. Once again it was the greatest meet ever held in America. The champions and their poundages follow:

THE CHAMPIONS OF 1933

112-POUND CLASS				
Lucien LaPlante, West End A. C., Gardner, Mass.	138	149	198.5	485.5
118-POUND CLASS				
Joe Fiorito, York Oil Burner A. C.	149	154.5	193	496.5
126-POUND CLASS				
Art Levan, York Oil Burner A. C.	160	176	231.5	568
132-POUND CLASS				
Mike Fontana, Lion Tailors, Akron, O.	165.5	176.5	237	579

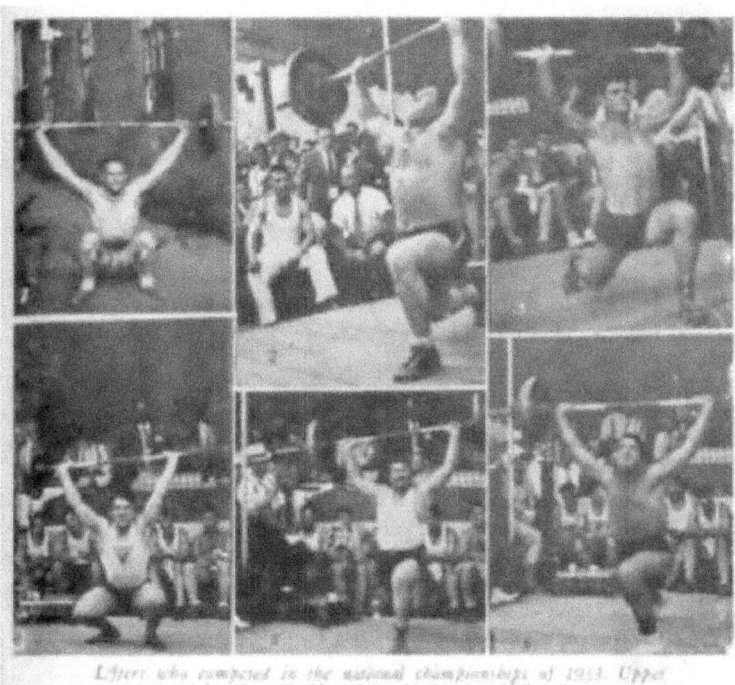

Lifters who competed in the national championships of 1933. Upper row, left to right—Bob Markley, John Mallo, Joe Miller. Lower row—Weldon Bullock, John Hice, George Mansur.

In John Mallo, America had a really big heavyweight for the first time—a man of the European type. Unfortunately an operation for appendicitis became necessary before a year had passed, and his strength was so great that he could not be controlled by the male nurses and doctors at the hospital as he was coming out of the ether, and he put up such a struggle that it resulted in his death.

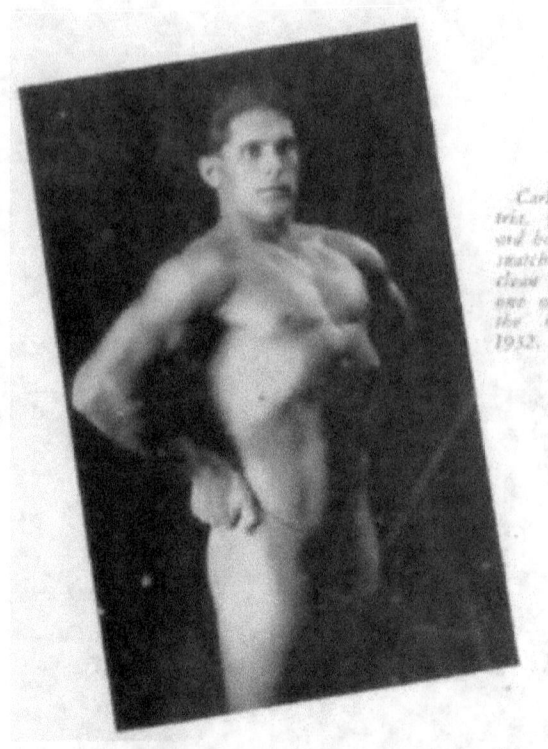

Carl Hipfinger, of Austria, former world's record holder in the left hand snatch and the two hands clean and jerk. He was one of the contestants in the Olympic games of 1932.

1932 was Olympic year, and for the first time in many years this quadrennial event was to be held in the United States. Los Angeles was the site of the games. This gave the United States an opportunity to compete internationally for the first time. Tryouts were held in various sections of the country, notably in Philadelphia, Detroit and Los Angeles and the best team we could put forth was selected. Dick Bachtell and Tony Terlazzo were the 132-pound lifters, Walk Zagurski and Amie Sundberg ihe lightweights. Stanley Kratkowski and Sam Termine of Los Angeles Athletic Club were the 165-pound men. Bill Good and Henry Dewey of Detroit the light-heavies, with Al Manger and Howard Turbifill as the heavyweights. These latter men were really light-heavies, just over the class limit, and could not be expected to compete on equal terms with the great European heavyweights.

36

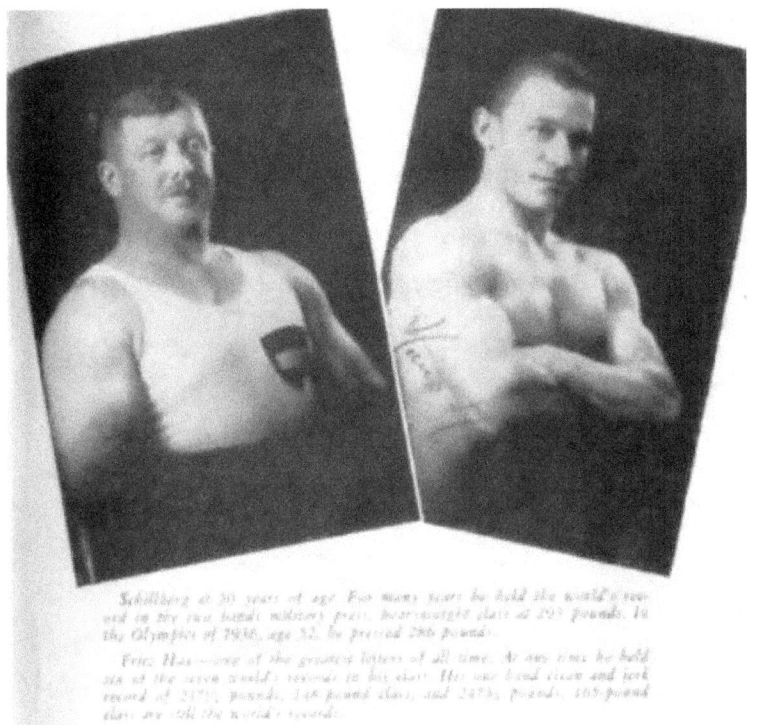

Schillbürg at 30 years of age. Two many years he held the world's record on the two hand military press, heavyweight class at 293 pounds. In the Olympics of 1936, age 32, he pressed 286 pounds.

Fritz Hau—one of the greatest lifters of all time. At one time he held six of the seven world's records to his class. His one hand clean and jerk record of 217½ pounds, 148-pound class, and 247½ pounds, 165-pound class are still the world's records.

At this stage of American weight lifting our men had not advanced to the point of being a serious threat in international weight lifting. Little did our lifters, the spectators or the foreign lifters, who looked upon the United States team as something of a joke, realize that in a few short years America was to have the world's strongest team.

As things turned out, Tony Terlazzo was the only American to defeat foreign lifters, finishing third in the 132-pound class. He made a valiant attempt with a double body weight clean and jerk which, had it been successful, would have brought him the title. The United States lifters gained experience; it gave me an opportunity to compare our lifting styles and training methods with the world's best lifters, and to note that we were on the right track.

In 1934 the five lifts were the basis for determining the nation's champion lifters. The championships that year were held at Ridgewood Grove, Brooklyn, N.Y. There were several upsets that year owing to the different set of lifts being employed—most notable of which was the failure of Tony Terlazzo to win a national title any year since his first national victory of 1932. He missed his three attempts on one of the lifts which permitted Bob Mitchell, also of the York team, to slip through and garner the title.

THE CHAMPIONS OF 1934

112-POUND CLASS
R. F. Knodle,
Hagerstown, Md. 88 132 154½ 132 187 693

118-POUND CLASS
Ralph Viera,
New Bedford, Mass... 99 120½ 148½ 154 203½ 731

126-POUND CLASS
Art Levan,
York Oil Burner A. C. 121 148½ 154 176 231 830½

132-POUND CLASS
Dick Bachtell,
York Oil Burner A. C. 143 159½ 170½ 181½ 242 896½

148-POUND CLASS
Bob Mitchell,
York Oil Burner A. C. 154 176 187 209 264 990

165-POUND CLASS
Stanley Kratkowski,
Detroit, Mich. 170½ 198 187 220 264 1039½
Gino Quilici,
Portland, Ore. 159½ 165 187 214½ 286 1012

HEAVYWEIGHT CLASS
Bill Good,
York, Pa. 192½ 220 225 247½ 324 1210

The championships of 1935 journeyed out to the southern Ohio city, Cincinnati. There they were ably conducted by Emmet Faris, long an enthusiastic lifter and weight lifting official. Joe Fiorito regained the championship lost the previous year at Brooklyn. Anthony Terlazzo came back to lead the lifters in the 148-pound class, while Wally Zagurski, who the previous year had lifted second to Kratkowski in the 163-pound class, yet making a higher total than the winner of the 181-pound class, had moved up. Again lie was unfortunate as he insisted on jumping on his second attempt on the one hand clean and jerk after the first attempt registered a failure. Two more failures and he was out, while a success with his first poundage would have given him the title as things turned out.

Complete report of the 1935 championships follows:

SENIOR NATIONAL CHAMPIONS OF 1935

	1 H. Snatch	1 H. C. & J	2 H. M. P.	2 H. Snatch	2 H. C. & J	Total
112-POUND CLASS						
David Rothman (N. Y.)	99	115½	132	115½	176	638
118-POUND CLASS						
Joe Fiorito (York)	104½	132	154	154	203½	718
126-POUND CLASS						
Art Levan (York)	132	137½	159½	176	236½	841½
132-POUND CLASS						
Dick Bachtell (York)	148½	176	170	181½	253	935
148-POUND CLASS						
Anthony Terlazzo (York)	159½	170½	209	203½	264	1006½
165-POUND CLASS						
Stanley Kratkowski (Detroit)	176	203½	181½	236½	297	1094½
181-POUND CLASS						
Steve Weisch (Newark)	170½	159½	192½	220	280½	1023½
HEAVYWEIGHT CLASS						
Bill Good (York)	192½	203½	231	247½	374½	1197

39

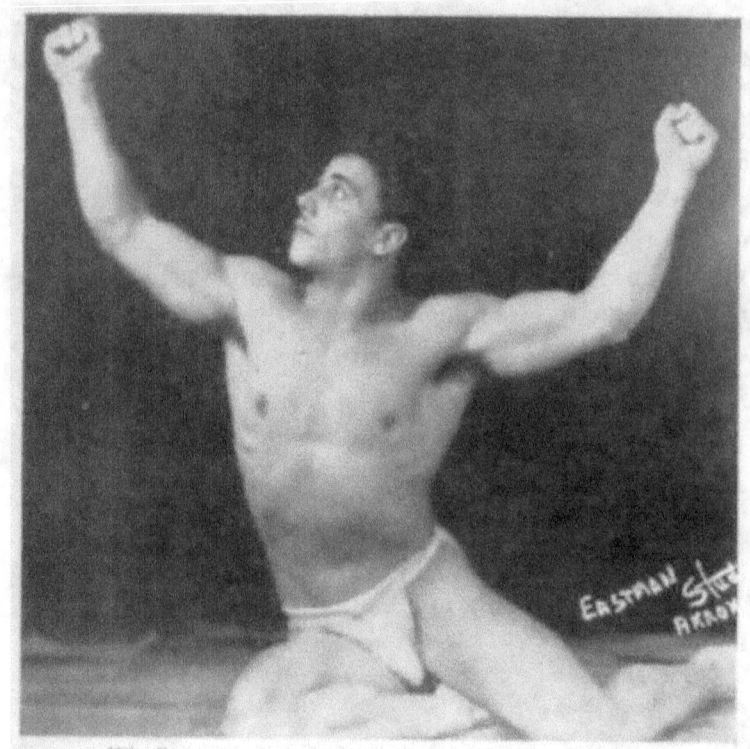

Mike Fontana—one of the best built men in America. He was the junior national champion at his weight, in 1943.

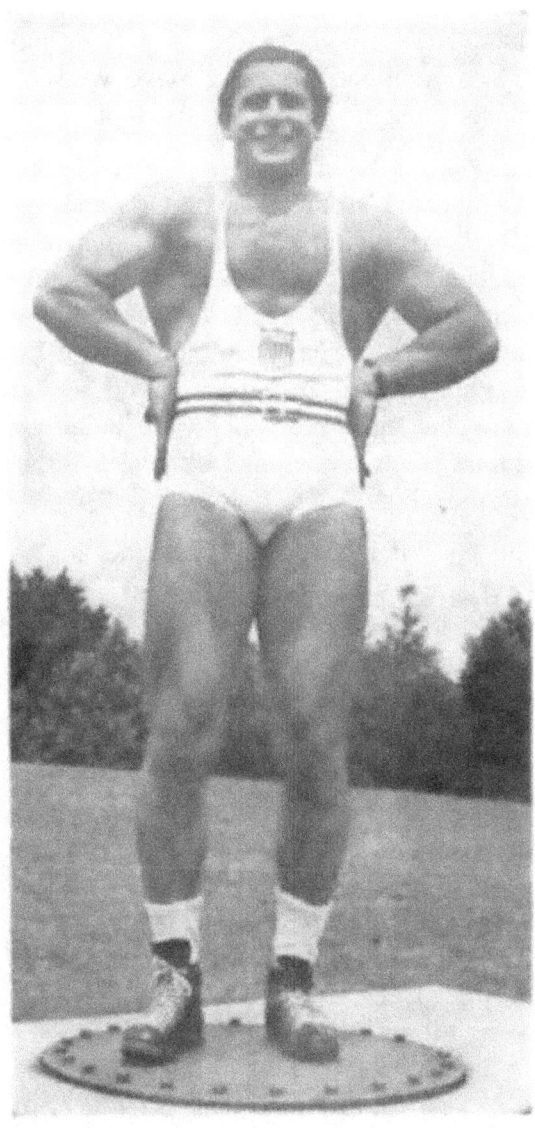

A close study of the records as compared to the previous year will illustrate that American lifting continued to rise. The perennial champions, Art Levan and Dick Bachtell, increased their totals on the five lifts by 11 and 39 pounds respectively. Terlazzo lifted 16 pounds more than the previous year's winner. Kratkowski hoisted 55 pounds more than in his victory of the preceding year. Steve Weisch of Prudential Insurance came up from his third place total with a gain of 50 pounds.

Once again as 1936 came around it was Olympic year. American lifting had been gaining to the point where our men closely approached the European standards in some of the body weight classes—notably in the featherweight and lightweight divisions. The national championships of 1936 were decided in Philadelphia and they served as final Olympic tryouts. As the three lifts only were being contested in the Olympics the two one hand lifts were dropped for that year's championships.

The most startling part of the program was the amazing lifting of Tony Terlazzo, who in winning the 132-pound title established a world's best press record of 215 pounds which has not been equalled to this day, nor has his lifting total of G93 been equalled by even the present world's title holder. The 1936 championships marked the first national senior victory for Johnny Terpak of York, who was destined to win the world's title the following year. A comparison of the clean and jerk records of the winners of this year, as compared to the previous year, illustrates a continued rise in United States lifting. In the classes starting with the 112, the first figures to be given represent the championship lifts of 1935, the second of 1936. The comparisons are as follows: 112-pound class, 176—176; 118-pound class, 203-209; 126-pound class, 236½ -242; 132-pound class, 253-269; 148-pound class, 264-297; 165-pound class, 297-302 ½; 181-pound class, 281-310.

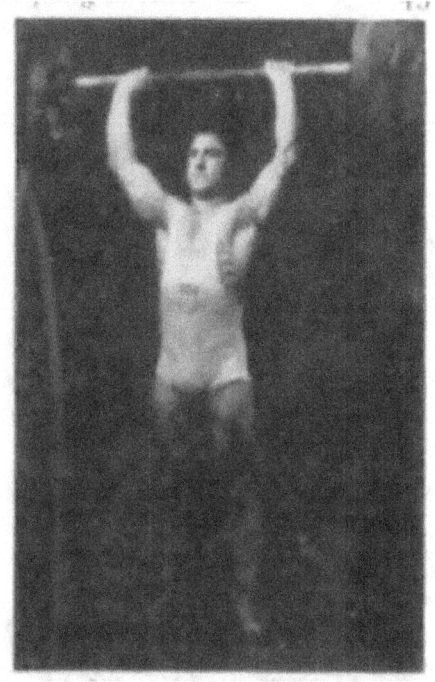

New records set that year were Fiorito's two hands snatch of 165, his two hands clean and jerk of 215 pounds; Art Levan's two hands snatch of 182, his clean and jerk of 242 pounds; the two hands press of 259[1] - of John Grimek in the heavyweight class, and the world's record of 215 made by Terlazzo in the 132-pound class.

The Olympic team was selected as follows: 132-pound men Terlazzo and John Terry; 148-pound class—Johnny Terpak and Bob Mitchell; 165-pound class Stanley Kratkowski and Walter Good; 181-pound class—Joe Miller and Bill Good; heavyweight class—John Grimek and Dave Mayor. Nine had been members of the York team. All were coached by myself.

SENIOR NATIONAL CHAMPIONS OF 1936

	Press	Snatch	Jerk	Total
112-POUND CLASS				
John Feitshe (Phila.)	137½	143	176	456½
118-POUND CLASS				
Joe Fiorito (York)	159½	165	209	533½
126-POUND CLASS				
Art Levan (York)	165	181½	242	588½
132-POUND CLASS				
Anthony Terlazzo (York)	214½	209	269½	693
148-POUND CLASS				
John B. Terpak (York)	220	220	297	737
165-POUND CLASS				
Stanley Kraikowski (Detroit)	214½	231	302½	748
181-POUND CLASS				
Joe Miller (York)	231	220	310	761
HEAVYWEIGHT CLASS				
John Grimek (York)	258½	220	308	786½

The 1936 Olympic team, left to right, sitting—Walter Good, Tony Terlazzo, John Terry, Bob Mitchell, John Grimek. Standing—A. A. U. national weight lifting chairman, Dietrich Wortmann, Joe Miller, Bill Good, Dave Mayor, Stanley Kraikowski and Johnny Terpak.

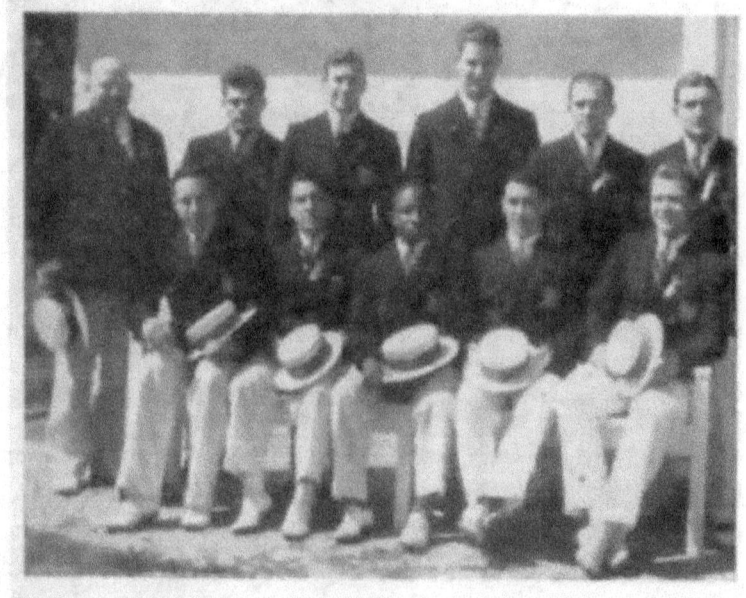

44

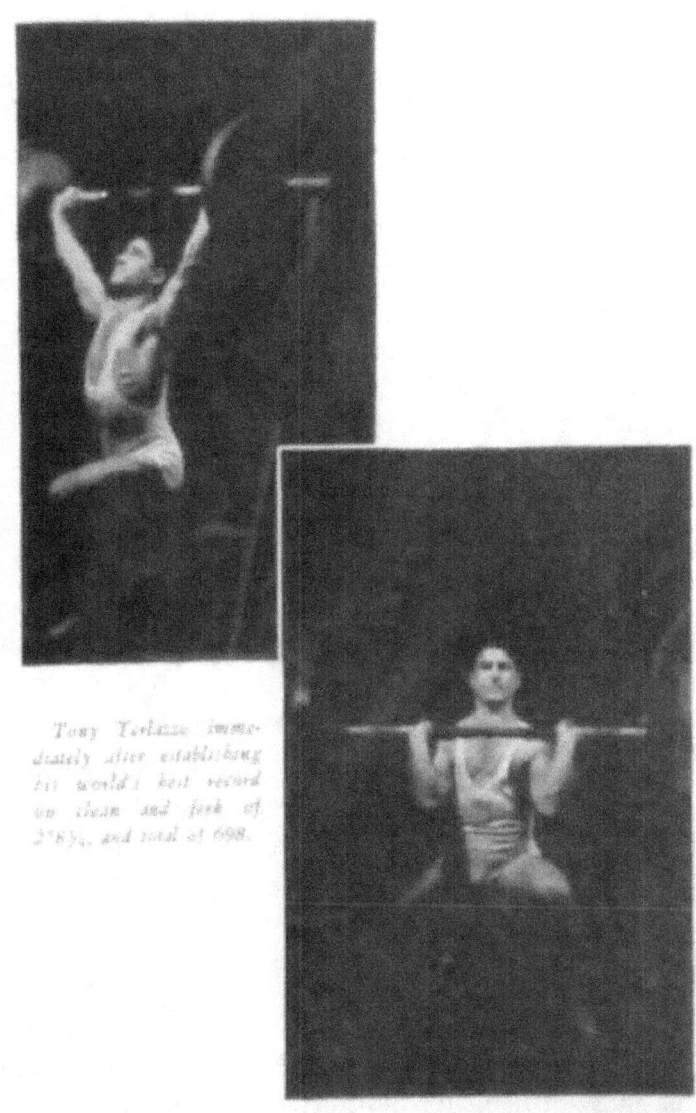

Tony Terlazzo imme-
diately after establishing
his world's best record
on clean and jerk of
325¾, and total of 698.

Although Strength and Health magazine had been published for some years and was finding its way to all corners
of the world, lifters and lifting officials in other countries
did not take American weight lifting seriously. But the
competition at Berlin proved to the lifting world that at last
the United States team had arrived and would be a factor in

future competition. Terlazzo came through beautifully to win the first world's title for America. He easily outclassed the remainder of the world's lifters, clinching the title with his first two hands clean and jerk. Terry, the powerful and beautifully built colored boy, the other lifter in the 132-pound class, finished among the place winners, making a clean and jerk of 264 pounds— double his body weight.

In the 148-pound class our lifters did not reach their previous best but Terpak finished among the place winners as did Kratkowski in the 165. Bill Good was among the point winners in the 181-pound class, although falling well behind his previous best totals. Grimek, the first American to finish in the heavyweight class, little more than a light-heavy, looked small compared to the mastodon-like European heavyweights and finished eighth. The American team as a whole scored in nearly every class and amassed a point score which won third place for them as a team. Of all the world's lifters, only Germany and Egypt, who put up a terrific battle for first place, succeeded in outscoring them.

1937 saw the senior national A.A.U. championships being decided in Wyandotte, Mich., al the fine, club house of the Michigan Alkali Club. For the first time lifters from Canada won titles in the United States national championships, Andy Hutchinson winning in the 112, and Eddie Hefferman in the 118. Both of these lifters were from Toronto. Art Levan for the first time abdicated his throne as champion of the 126-pound class- a championship that he had held for ten consecutive years. Each year it had become increasingly difficult for him to reduce to the 126- pound class, and this year of 1937 he competed in the 148- pound division, where he was outclassed by normally larger and heavier men.

The most notable improvement during this year was 011 the part of Terlazzo and Terpak, the former amassing the amazing total of 780 to shatter the world's record in his class for a total on the three lifts. The Olympic winners in that division had scored 753 as compared to Terlazzo's 780 in our national championships. Johnny Terpak scored 805, a total that had only been officially surpassed by one man—that being Touni, the marvelous Olympic 165-pound champion. His clean and jerk of 325 pounds, especially notable as his body weight was but 158, gained him national fame. The performance of these two York lifters was a good forecast of their victories in their classes at the world's championships held later that year in Paris. Dave Mayor who had competed in the Olympics made the highest total of the championships to win his first senior national title.

We will compare the total of the three lifts made by the winners of 1936 and 1937: 112-pound class, 456-515; 118-pound class, 533ˉ535; 126-pound class, 588-585; 132-pound class, 693-635; 148-pound class, 737-780 —a substantial gain of 43 pounds as Terlazzo moved back into the 148-pound class to win the championship vacated by Johnny Terpak and in the 165, Stanley Kratkowski's winning total of 744 was stretched to 805 by Johnny Terpak; 181-pound class, 761-800; heavyweight, 786 ¼—835.

	Press	Snatch	Jerk	Total
112-POUND CLASS				
Andy Hutchinson (Toronto)	155	160	200	515
118-POUND CLASS				
Ed Hefferman (Toronto)	160	165	210	535
126-POUND CLASS				
Michael Mungioli (Maspeth, L. I.)	165	195	225	585
132-POUND CLASS				
Dick Bachtell (York)	185	200	250	635
148-POUND CLASS				
Anthony Terlazzo (York)	235	240	305	780
165-POUND CLASS				
John Terpak (York)	235	245	325	805
181-POUND CLASS				
Bill Good (Reamstown)	235	240	325	800
HEAVYWEIGHT CLASS				
Dave Mayor (York)	250	255	330	835

The world's championships of 1937 were to be contested in Paris, so it was decided to send a team. Each club was to pay the way of the men who represented them. The first and second place winners in each class were eligible for the trip. As the team was selected, I arranged the finances for our own four champions—Bachtell, Terlazzo, Terpak and Mayor—and sent Venables along as competing manager and 181-pound class man. The Raymond A. C. of Cleveland paid the transportation for Joe Germ, featherweight; German-American A. C. of New York Dietrich Wortmann's club—for John Terlazzo, 148-pound lifter, member of that club and brother of Tony Terlazzo, the great York champion.

Terlazzo did what lifting experts throughout the world said he could not do—won the title in the 148-pound class. The previous year his Olympic title had been won at 132 and here he was, a full-fledged 148-pounder, good enough to gain the world's title, and he had to break his world's total record to win—and then only by 5 ½ pounds —over Fein, the Austrian lightweight. Terlazzo equalled the world's record in the two hands snatch and set a new world mark in the clean and jerk, his record being 315 pounds. Terpak surprised by winning the world's 165-pound title. Travelling conditions and living conditions were not of the best. Our entire team was ill during much of the crossing, and failed to do their best. but two titles out of five were something to be elated about. The United States had really arrived as a world lifting power. Once again our team finished third, this time back of Germany and Austria.

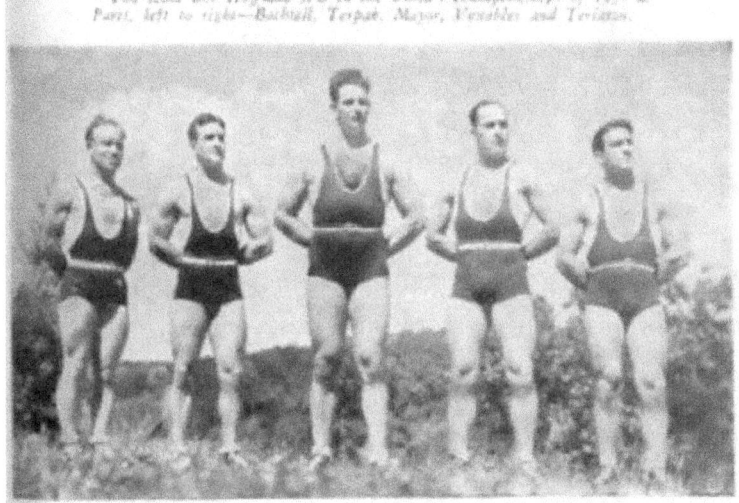

The team Bob Hoffman sent to the world's championships of 1937 at Paris, left to right—Bachtell, Terpak, Mayor, Venables and Terlazzo.

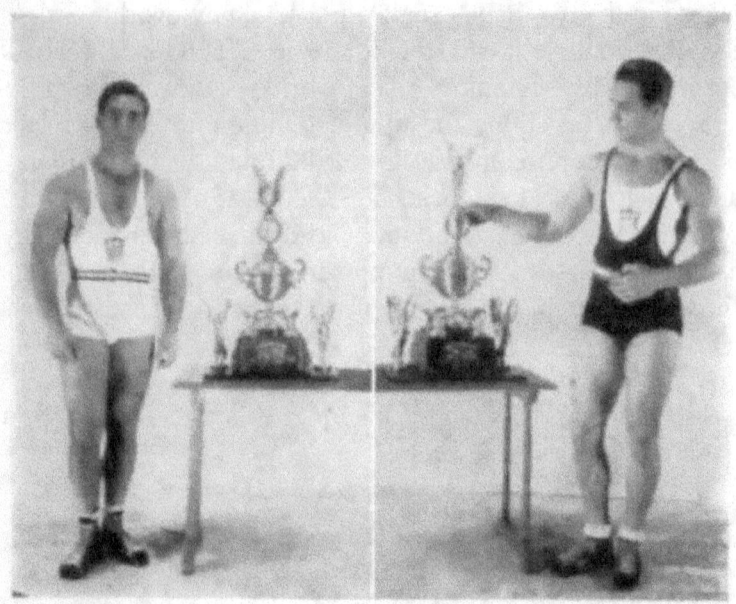

Then came 1938, a year which was destined to provide still more thrills and still more surprises in American lifting. New stars were to rise and overshadow those of the past. The two biggest surprises were John "Hercules" Davis and Steve Stanko. Stanley Kratkowski registered splendid improvement, scoring a fine 805. To win his title he broke the American record on the last lift with a hoist of 330 pounds. Never were there so many thrills, so much enthusiasm at a national championship. Stanko, an almost unheard-of lifter, competing at his third meet, broke his own record in the clean and jerk by fifteen pounds to win the national title by a scant five pounds. Complete summary of the lifting:

National Champions of 1938

	Press	Snatch	C. & J.	Total
112-Pound Class				
A. Lemma	205	145	210	560
118-Pound Class				
B. Leardi	155	165	200	520
126-Pound Class				
M. Mungioli	175	185	240	600
132-Pound Class				
J. Terry	170	205	265	640
148-Pound Class				
A. Terlazzo	220	225	320	765
165-Pound Class				
J. Terpak	235	250	300	785
181-Pound Class				
S. Kratkowski	225	250	330	805
Heavyweight Class				
S. Stanko	245	260	345	850

National Champions of 1939

	Press	Snatch	C. & J.	Total
112-Pound Class				
A. Firpo Lemma	195	130	205	530
118-Pound Class				
Bill Leardi	150	165	210	525
126-Pound Class				
Elwrod P. Caufmann	155	180	225	560
132-Pound Class				
John Terry	185	215	260	660
148-Pound Class				
Anthony Terlazzo	250	245	310	805
165-Pound Class				
John Terpak	235	240	325	800
181-Pound Class				
John Davis	255	260	300	815
Heavyweight Class				
Steve Stanko	270	280	345	895

123-POUND CLASS				
Joe Fiorito	160	170	220	550
132-POUND CLASS				
John Terry	185	210	270	665
148-POUND CLASS				
Tony Terlazzo	240	230	300	770
165-POUND CLASS				
John Terpak	240	235	325	800
181-POUND CLASS				
John Davis	250	275	330	855
HEAVYWEIGHT CLASS				
Steve Stanko	290	300	360	950

NATIONAL CHAMPIONS OF 1941

123-POUND CLASS				
Wesley Cochrane	175	190	250	615
132-POUND CLASS				
John Terry	190	205	270	665
148-POUND CLASS				
Anthony Terlazzo	250	240	310	800
165-POUND CLASS				
John Terpak	245	250	320	815
181-POUND CLASS				
Frank Kay	265	260	325	850
HEAVYWEIGHT CLASS				
John Davis	320	315	370	1005

A world's championship team contest was to take place in 1938. The German team, Olympic and world's team champions, numbering three world's champions on their roster and the men who held fully half of the world's records, expressed a willingness to come here to lift against our team. The German team consisted of George Liebsch, world's 132-pound champion, Carl Jansen, former European champion in the 148-pound class, Rudi Ismayr,

Olympic and world's champion of previous years, Tony Gietl, world's record holder in the 181-pound class, and Joseph Manger, Olympic and world's heavyweight champion.

Our own team included the national champions of 1938— John Terry, Tony Terlazzo, Johnny Terpak, Stanley Kratkowski and Steve Stanko. The contest was held in the city of Baltimore, June 19th, before a big crowd. The United States won three of the classes, with Terlazzo, Terpak and Kratkowski outscoring their men. On the basis of points, the United States team won. Counting the poundages elevated to arm's length overhead, the German team were victors by 38 pounds. It was a close contest, with the teams finishing less than one per cent apart. Had Johnny Davis been a bit farther advanced and scored the same total he made later in winning his world's title—853—the United States team would have won this great international match. But it was an honor and credit to our team to be lifting against, on an equal basis, the great European champions and world's record holders who were formerly almost legendary figures to us. The superiority of Manger in two hands pressing, as compared to our own young champion, Steve Stanko (236 against 302 — 66 pounds), was much more than the margin of victory of the German team.

Right now, with continued improvement on the part of all of our lifters, with sensational gains by Davis and Stanko, America has the strongest team in the world. Yes, stronger than Germany and Austria combined. Austria placed second in Paris you may remember, and even with the addition of the Czecho-Slovakian team, who have Olympic, world's and European champions among them, we still have the world's strongest team. But more about that later.

The world's championships of 1938 were scheduled for Vienna, and there was so much agitation and excitement, so much threat of war, battle almost a certainty at times, that our lifters could not know until the last minute whether there were to be championships or not. But finally it was decided to send the team. I furnished their transportation but pressure of business did not permit me to make the trip. Donna Fox, long an athletic enthusiast, co-winner of the two-man bob sled championship at the Olympics of 1936, was their manager and ably handled the job.

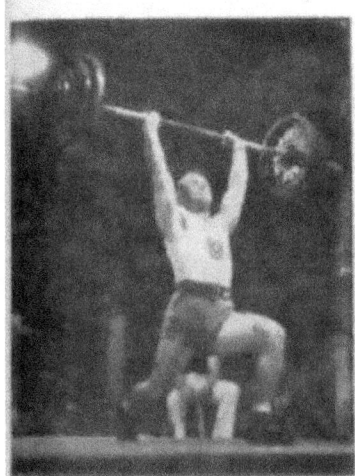 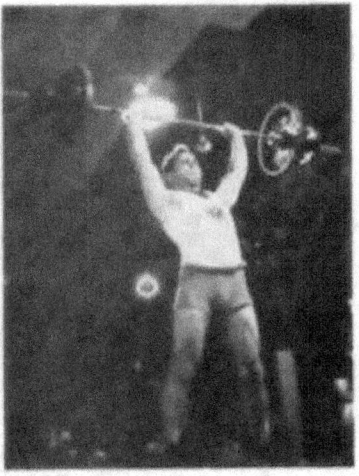

Upper left Carl Jansen, German 148 pound champion and former European champion. Upper right Tony Gitel, world's record holder 181 pound class, two hands military press. Below—Rudi Ismayr, Olympic champion of 1932, world's champion other years. At one time or other held all the world's middleweight records. He was captain of the German team which competed with the U. S. team in our country during 1938.

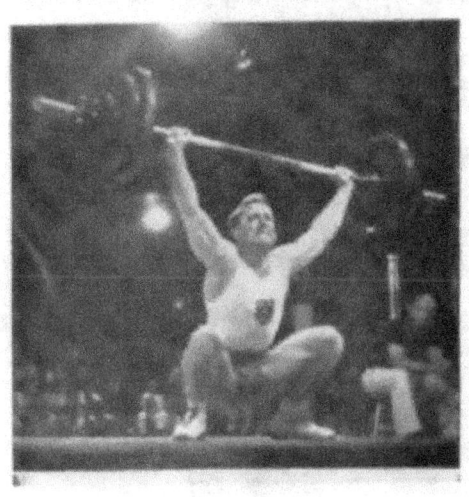

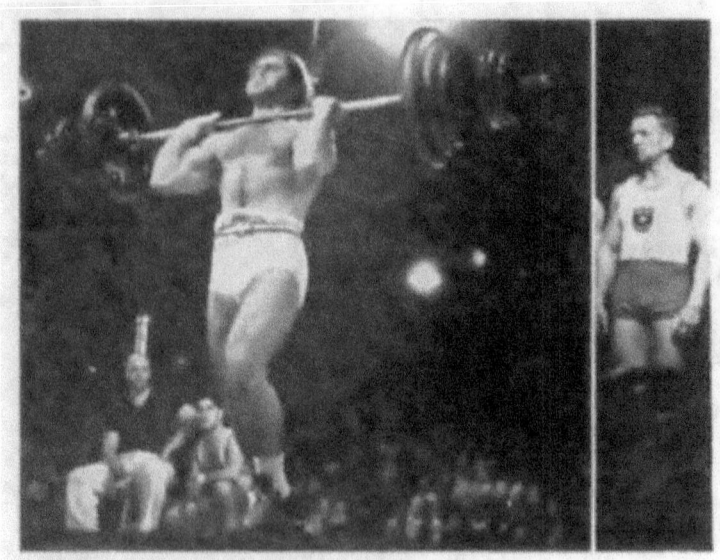

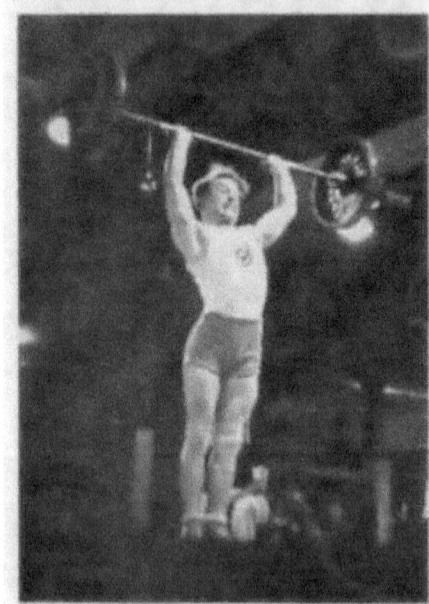

Upper left—Steve Stanko successfully cleaning 350 pounds. At left—George Liebisch, world's champion 132-pound class.

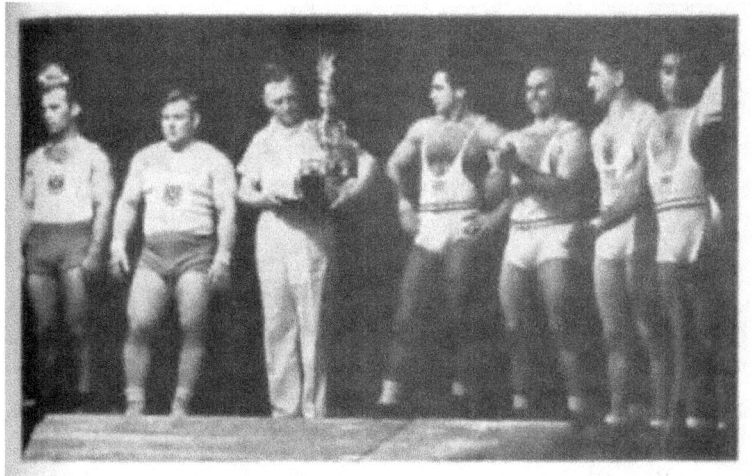

The United States and German teams at the time of their world's championship team match in Baltimore, June 19, 1938. The German team's manager is holding the Bob Hoffman trophy which was presented to the German team.

Final trials were held to be sure that all lifters had maintained their previous form. The trials staged at Toronto showed great improvement on the part of Grimek, as he and John Davis both outscored Kratkowski, the national 181-pound champion, and made the team. Terry, the 132-pound champion, Terlazzo and Terpak, respectively champions in the 148 and 165, and Stanko, the heavyweight champion, made up the team.

And once again they failed to win the world's team championship by a small margin. Terry finished third in his class, establishing a new world's record in the two hands snatch. The officials turned down his presses so he had too bad a start to hope to win. Terlazzo won his third world's title this time, staving off the rush of the great Egyptians as well as the European lifters. Johnny Terpak, although lifting more than he did the previous year, failed to repeat. The officials turned down his press which placed him in a bad spot. In the clean and jerk he made too big a jump from his first success with 308 to 330 which was more than lie could hope to succeed with after a very long wait—a stormy trip across the ocean with no lifting equipment to train with. Making a mighty effort to win permitted Ismayr to come through for second place and there went our chances to win.

But John Davis, not yet eighteen years of age, was to startle the world with a victory in the 181-pound class, defeating the great former champions—Hostin of France, and Haller, formerly of Austria. Grimek finished fourth and was capable of making a higher total. He had enough to beat the lifters but the officials used some mysterious methods in this class. Grimek's perfect snatch of 253 was turned down, while Hala of Germany, the expected winner, was permitted to press out the weight and remain for some seconds with his knee touching the platform. In the heavy-weight division, Stanko certainly did all that could be expected by winning second place, making the highest two hands snatch and the highest clean and jerk of any of the world's lifters. Our lifters finished second by a slender margin.

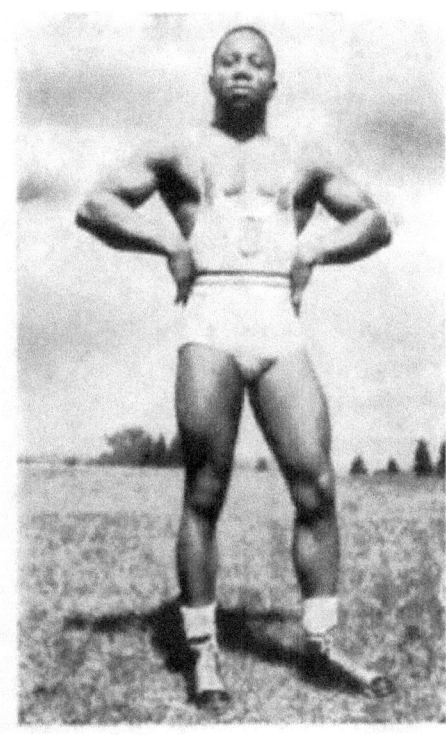

John Terry, famous York lifter, member of the 1936 Olympic team, holder of the world's record in the two hands snatch 132-pound class at 215 pounds, the world's record in the dead weight lift at 585 pounds, national champion of 1938, member of the world's championship teams and a place winner both at Berlin and Vienna.

So the American team right now is up at the top the world's strongest team, figuring oil the basis of recent performances. Recently Terlazzo and Davis have shattered world's records, Terlazzo breaking the world's press record by a full eight and a half pounds, equalling the world's clean and jerk record, while John Davis shattered the former world's mark in the two hands press by a full 22 pounds. Only one pound is required to break a world's record and this feat is unprecedented. He also surpassed the world's record in the clean and jerk by a small margin, pushing the world's record in the total of the three lifts to new heights. And Stanko is getting better every day and is closely approaching world's records in the two hands snatch and the two hands clean and jerk, while his press record is constantly rising.

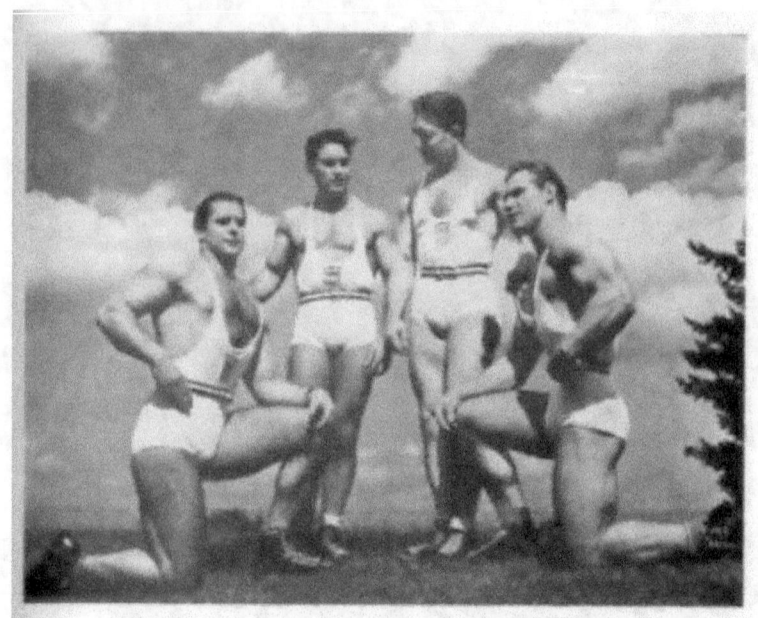

Four All-American lifters of 1938—Steve Stanko, United States heavyweight champion; Tony Terlazzo, Olympic, world's and national champion; Johnny Terpak, world's and national champion; John Grimek, champion of North America.

At present the records of our five best men as compared to the best German quintet are as follows:

George Liebsch	681
Karl Jansen	753
Adolph Wagner	814
Fritz Haller	830
Joseph Manger	946
John Terry	675
Tony Terlazzo	835
John Terpak	845
John Davis	901
Steve Stanko	1020

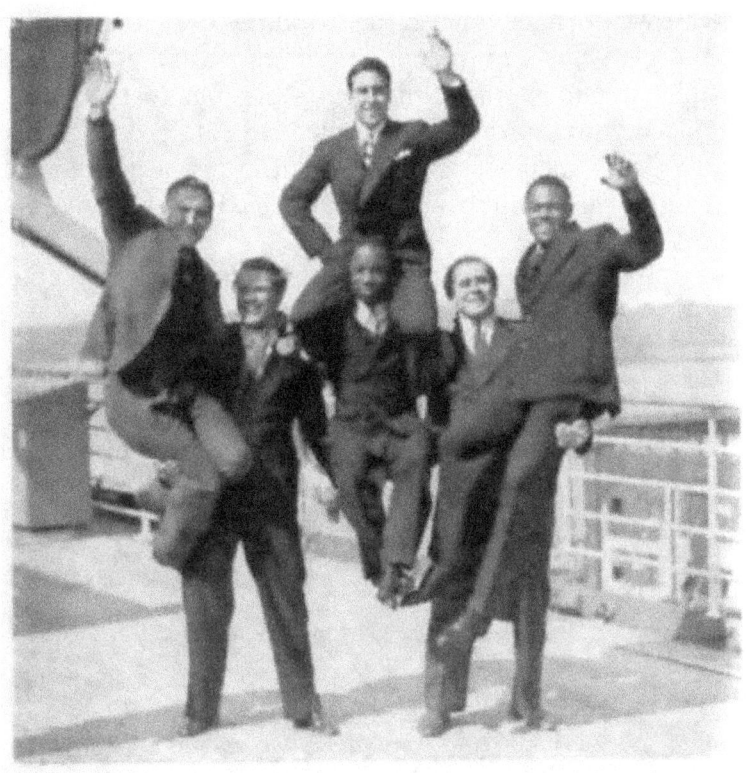

The American team the writer sent to Vienna to compete in the world's championship. Terlazzo and 17-year-old John Davis won world's titles. Left to right—Terpak, Gismek, Terry, Terlazzo, Stanko and Davis.

We have traced the rise of American weight lifting to the point where it leads the world. Owing to the war there were no official world's championships in weight lifting during 1939-1940-1941. In the years before the war American lifters advanced to the point where Terlazzo, Terpak and Davis scored victories in the 148, 165 and 181-pound classes respectively, with Stanko second in the heavyweight and Terry third in the 132. The improvement of our men has been so sensational that it is reasonable to believe that with fair officiating they would win the five championships or official world's championships, if they were held at present. One of the great difficulties our lifters had to overcome was European officials in whose eyes their own men can never be wrong—while those from across the water can seldom be right. We have proven that in this country we have the men - that our (or perhaps I should say my, for all of these men have been coached by me) training methods are right, so it is just a question of time until we definitely and officially lead the world weight lifters.

Winners of the first three places in the world's championships of 1938. Terlazzo the winner, Attia of Egypt second and Schmidt of Germany third.

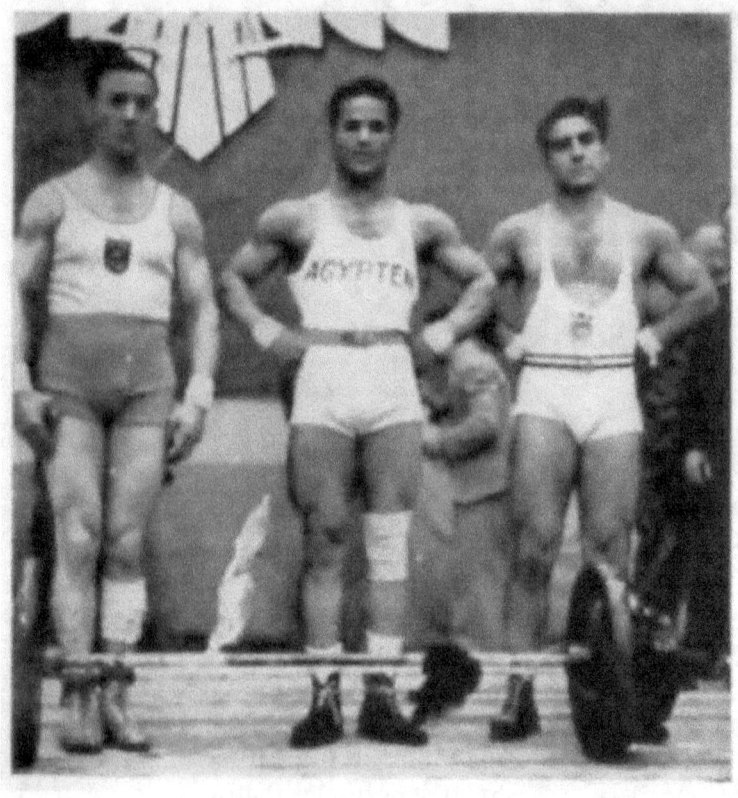

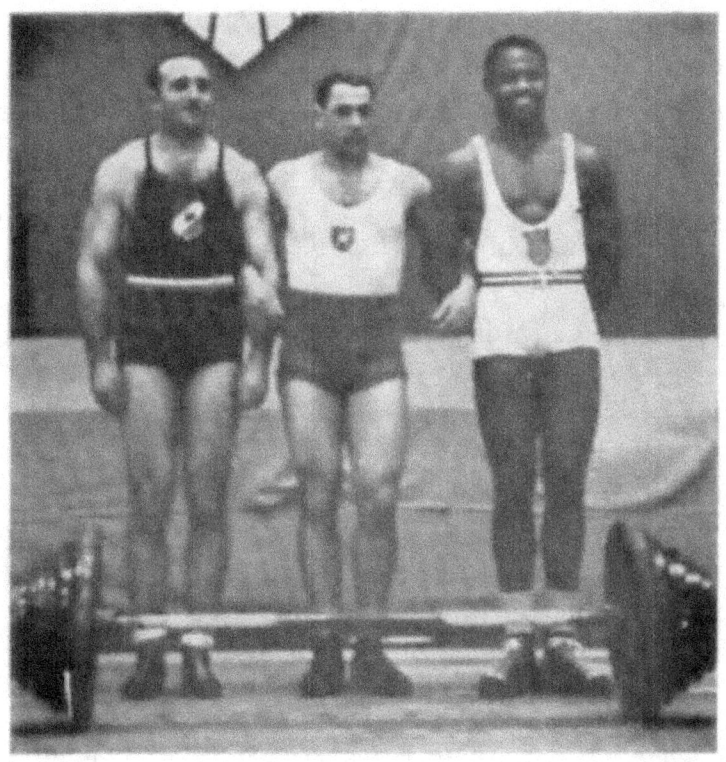

The winners in the 181-pound class at Vienna. Left to right—Hostin of France, Olympic champion in 1932 and 1936, who finished third; Haller of Austria world's champion of 1937, world's record holder two hands snatch, who finished second; and John Davis of the York team, who won the world's title.

Champions I Have Trained

Close perusal of the championship results throughout the years will disclose that a majority of the championships have been won by representatives of our team. At present all of the records- three lifts and totals, in the five Olympic body weight classes, twenty in all—are held by members of the York team. It's natural that interested persons should wonder just how York became the world center for this sport of weight lifting, just why America's strongest men usually find their way to York, later to win world-wide weight lifting acclaim. So I'll start at the beginning and tell you something of my own team.

In another chapter I briefly mentioned that I first learned of weight lifting in 1923. Before that year I had. from as early as I could remember, a desire to be stronger than the average physically and to excel at athletics. I had practiced most every form of exercise and had good success with all popular branches of athletics. But I had been tall and thin to begin, narrow-shouldered and chicken-breasted, and although all the sports—rowing, canoeing, swimming, boxing, wrestling, gymnastics, handball, baseball, basketball, football, etc., etc.,—had played their part in building my physical ability to a certain extent, it seemed that I had not received improvement commensurate with the effort put forth and the time I had spent at all forms of physical training.

In addition to the athletic pastimes I have enumerated. I had followed "train you by mail systems" as early as at the age of ten years, if had tried light dumbells, cable exercisers, springs of all sorts, rowing machines, wall pulleys, calisthenics of every imaginable type. Hour after hour I had trained until the floor was wet with my perspiration. I frequently went to work tired completely, in spite of very unusual endurance, from my endeavors to get a body like the "train you by mail" professors whose courses I took, by following the system of exercises they offered.

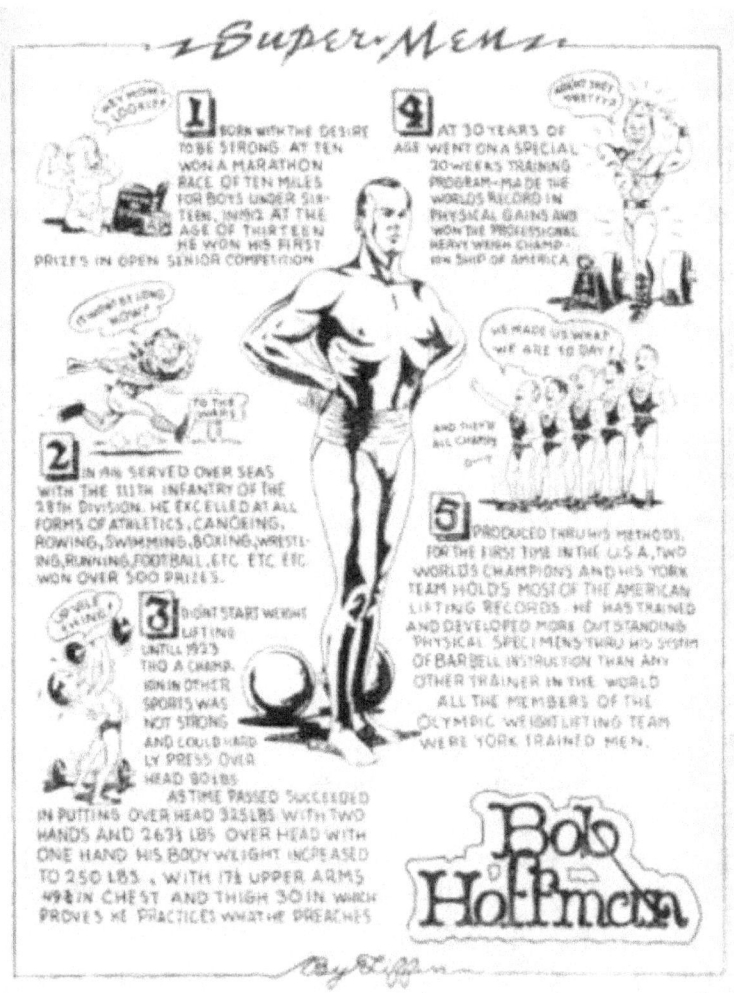

I had weighed 140 pounds when I first reached my height of six feet three inches. I had weighed 167 as a national champion before the war, and 180 after returning from France and reaching the age of 21—not much weight for my height. And in that year of 1923 I learned the apparently carefully guarded secret that the strong men became strong through weight training. But almost without exception, for profit reasons only (it being more profitable to sell a few printed pages than heavy weights—expensive to build, machine and pack), they offered courses with light apparatus or with no form of equipment. I tried all the systems and very little was obtained for my pains.

And then I learned about weight lifting, learned that that was the way all strong men worthy of the name had become strong. Weight lifting was an exercise that could be followed progressively—one that was suitable for the weakest man or woman, for such a person could start with as little as fifteen pounds if they preferred and work up in gradual increases of as little as a pound and a quarter at a time. As the strength increased more weight could be added.

After my introduction to weight lifting I became very enthusiastic concerning the sport and took advantage of every opportunity to engage in lifting contests, to visit weight lifting gymnasiums throughout the country, and to train with weight lifters in the city where I might be, as my work was travelling about fifty thousand miles a year. All of this experience and the great improvement in my own physical strength and athletic ability, my speed and endurance, the marvelous, pulsating, vibrating, thrilling health and strength I enjoyed, convinced me that weight lifting was the best body conditioner not only for those who wish to obtain the maximum of health, strength and development but for those athletes who desire to improve at their chosen sport.

During the earlier years of my acquaintance with and interest in weight lifting, I was an amateur athlete. I participated in amateur athletics for the pleasure it gave me and the favorable physical results it brought. It was my work to travel every week of the year to advance the business in which f was engaged. There came a time when intensive application to the manufacturing business in which I was a partner demanded so much of my time, long hours into the night, that I was forced to neglect my exercise. So I had the opportunity to learn just how it felt to possess "able to be around" health. I wasn't sick, but I didn't have much pep, after years of intensive work. I felt heavy on my feet and didn't have the appetite I once enjoyed. When my business had advanced to the point where I could spend much of the time in York I took the first opportunity to go back to weight training.

This was in the year 1930 and I was nearly 32 years of age at the time. In just seven weeks' time, from this rather average beginning, I became much stronger, better built, could lift more weight than ever before and once again enjoyed perfect health and energy. Others who were employed at the factory of which i was part owner—the York Oil Burner Company—saw the results I was obtaining and decided to try some of the same iron pills—weight training. Soon a group of us were training, and not long after that we received a challenge from a team in Hagerstown for a contest. The contest took place and we won by a small margin.

I remember that contest well. Our team at that time consisted of Art Levan, Joe Miller, who was a very powerful young man but with little lifting skill, the two Schell boys—Lou and Floyd—and myself. On the other team were Dick Bachtell and Bob Knodic, national champions, and Charles Snyder. I succeeded in making the highest lifts in the one hand snatch, the one hand clean and jerk, and the two hands jerk—145, 175 and 250 being my marks after a few weeks of training. Joe Miller made the highest press—185- and the highest two hands snatch—190.

The Hagerstown team improved, our team got better and better, we won three contests in a row by small margins. Soon we had become strong enough to lift against an All-Maryland team which included, besides the two national champions already on the team, the heavyweight national champion from Baltimore, Al Manger. We were able to win from the All-Maryland team. In contest after contest I made the highest clean and jerk—only 260 pounds -which according to present standards is not great, but was considered a heavy lift in those days, nearly a decade ago. Joe Miller was improving and soon gave me competition in the two hands clean and jerk. I could only lift 220 in that style in practice. Joe could make 290, yet in several contests we both succeeded with 260 pounds, I could outdo myself in competition. Joe would become nervous and not perform as well.

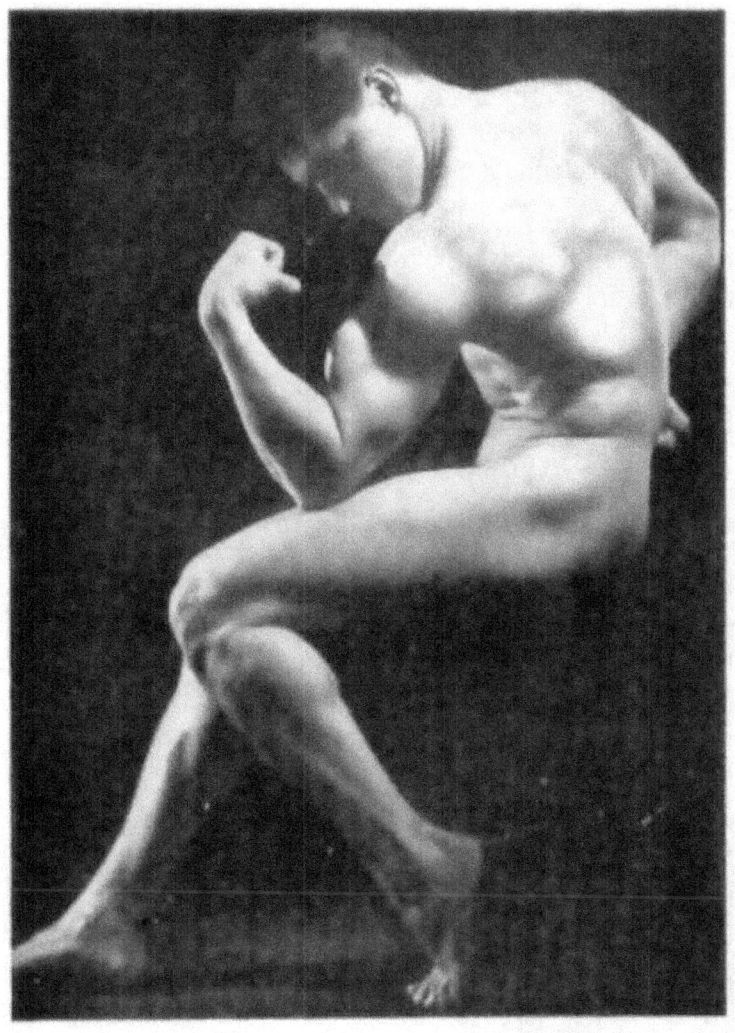

George Kichi of Chicago, a famous before and after case. In this photo he weighs 186. Through his hard training and lifting he increased his weight from 120 pounds.

Finally our team was attracting national attention and we received an invitation to lift against the national team champions of that year—German-American A. C. of New York. It was now the end of 1931 and we fondly hoped and believed that we had a team which could cope with the German-American on equal terms. But we were to be disillusioned. The All-Maryland team took part. The German-American team, made up of champions, former champions, German champions, was too much for our group of young men and we lost, although we did outlift the All-Maryland team.

In spite of the fact that five of the 1931 national United States champions were in action, once again the highest lift made was 260 pounds, this amount being hoisted by Hans Ehrhart, Steve Brodsky of German-American and myself.

Bill Good and Walter Good were present at this contest and they asked to be members of the team. Later their application was accepted.

We had a beautiful place in York, a private gymnasium, a club with showers, electric refrigeration, kitchen, beautiful lawns, shrubs and flowers and all who came here envied us our training facilities and equipment and wished to be a part of that club. Weight lifting had been a sport which was practiced in large measure in the back rooms of saloons, in barns or bedrooms, prior to this time, and for the first time weight lifting was being placed on a much higher plane.

Another match with German-American was scheduled. But in the meantime, returning from a weight lifting contest near Philadelphia January 3rd, 1932, we had a very severe accident. Our car which had cost 1900 dollars was so completely demolished that we left it on the hill. I was unconscious four days and although no bones were broken I experienced nerve injuries that arc still fell on occasional rainy days to this time. But 1 got up and around after a time. Weight lifters arc hard to kill, I guess. Our roadster had been hit with a car going sixty miles an hour, turned over and over where it burst into flame. Luckily my unconscious body was pulled from the car or, without being immodest, I believe it only fair to say that American weight lifting would not be where it is today.

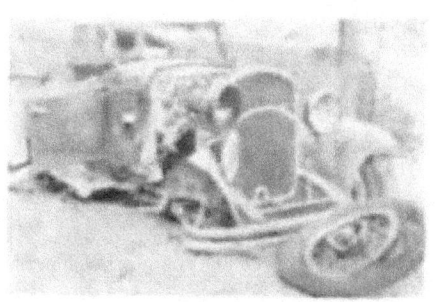

The wrecked car from which the author was fortunate enough to emerge alive.

I was not able to lift in the next contest but the addition of Bill and Walter Good, with Joe Miller, Art Levan, Joe Fiorito, Lou and Hooley Schell brought our team to the point where it lost by only a few pounds. We had been competing with German-American on a seven-man team basis, and as their smaller men outweighed ours considerably, it was decided that the next contest would include the five Olympic body weight classes only.

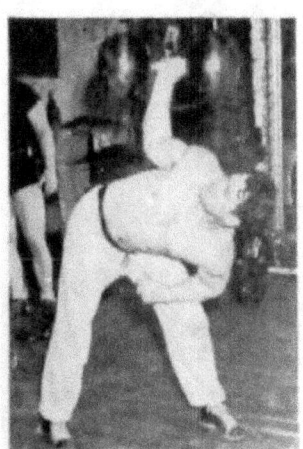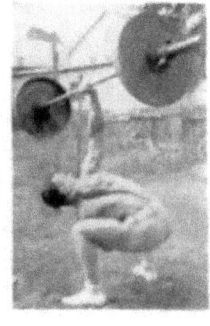

Wally Zagurski bent pressing the most famous piece of iron in the world, the Cyr bell, with which Louis Cyr, the strongest man who ever lived, broke Sandow's record with a lift of 273 pounds. In smaller illustration—Wal Di Genova, American lightweight bent press champion. He has lifted 60 pounds more than his body weight in this style.

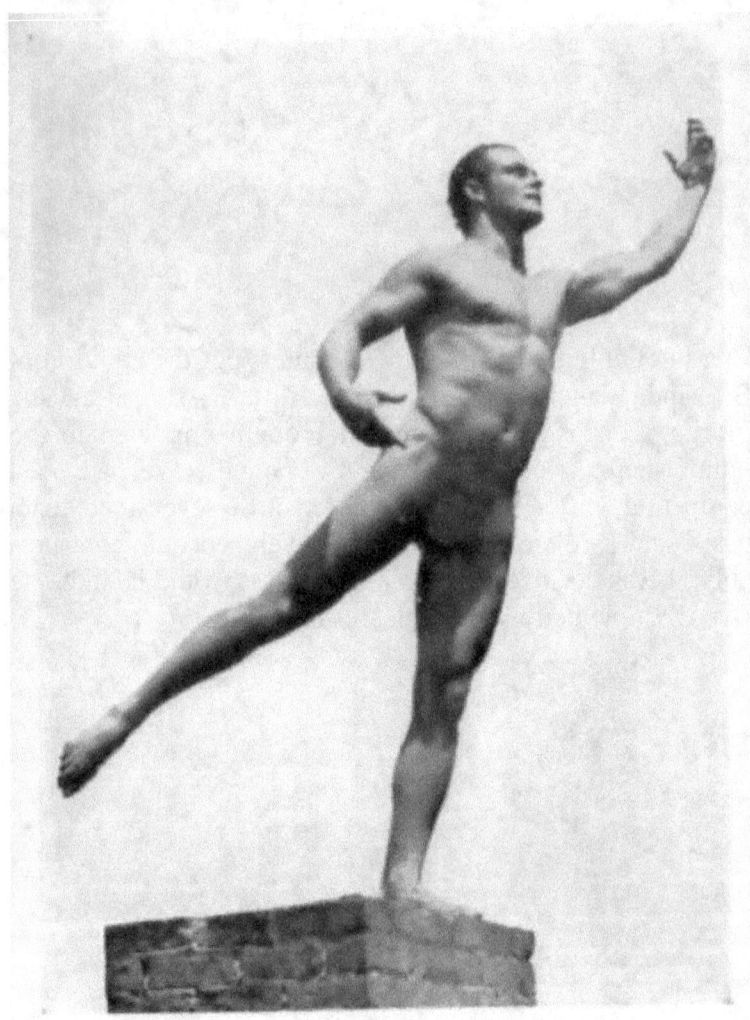

Bill Hillgardner of New York City, a York bar bell man, who has won renown for his development. Frequently the winner of physical excellence contests.

I encouraged all the members of our team, was teaching them lifting according to the style that I had found to behest—lifting methods that are identical with those we still use—and every man was improving rapidly. We expected to win this time for sure. And then just two days before the contest, we received a communication that not the club whose first team scored the highest number of points, but the club whose first and second team hoisted the greatest poundage would win the big silver cup and the gold medals. This put us on a real spot. We only had one team and an extra lifter or two. Dick Bachtell had been writing to me stating that he was so anxious to come to York that he would walk here on his hands and knees the entire seventy miles from Hagerstown if he could find work here. So 1 found a job for him. And Wally Zagurski who had been unemployed for two years had been writing to me. I phoned him and found work for him too. This gave us a second team with one of our factory employees, and myself as the heavyweight, still weak from my injuries.

Our team outdid themselves, lifted far more than ever before—with the exception of myself. I could press only 121 and clean and jerk 236, in my weakened condition. Strange as it may seem we won; defeated the national team champions for the first time. We have the big cup we won that day among many other trophies in our offices.

We had the national A.A.U. championships in York that year, and our York Oil Burner A. C. (our team represented the company in which I was part owner and president) became the national team champions—an honor that they won again last year for the seventh consecutive time. Our team at the nationals that year consisted of Dick Bachtell who tied for first in the 132-pound class; Joe Fiorito who won the 118-pound title; Harry Thomasiko who was second in the 112; Lou Schell, fourth in the 132; Joe Miller tied for first in the 165-pound class; George Brown, fourth in the 126-pound class; Art Levan, winner in the 126; Walter Good tied for third in the 181; Wally Zagurski, third in the 165; Bob Pent/., fourth in the 112; Reed Swartz, eighth in his class; Tony Maniscalco, fifth in the 148-pound class, and Bill Good, first in the 181.

A number of our men made the Olympic team- Bill Good, Dick Bachtell and Wally Zagurski. Before the Olympics

Tony Terlazzo had been living in York and after the Olympics being unable to find employment in or around New York or New Jersey, where his people lived, he came to York and found work.

There was much activity during that year of late 1932 and early 1933. And by the time of the national championships of 1933 we had a much improved team which lined up as follows: Wally Zagurski, first in the 165; Lou Schell, fourth in the 132; Anthony Fiorito, fourth in the 126; Gus Modiri, who that year won the 132-pound junior title, was third in the 132; Frank Tornetta was third in the 112; Walter Good, fourth in the 181; Joe Fiorito, first in the 118; Weldon Bullock, 17-year-old wonder, who made the meet's highest clean and jerk although finishing in fourth position in his class; Dick Bachtcll, second in the 132; Bill Good, lirst in the 181: Art Levari, first in the 126; Bob Mitchell, second in the 165; Tom Terlazzo, first in the 148; George Brown, third in the 126; and Joe Miller, second in the heavyweight division. The York Oil Burner A. C., in spite of two unexpected failures in the 132 and the heavyweight divisions, had amassed a total of 39 points to the second club's 11 and as compared to 35 for all other clubs.

It was a wonderful team.

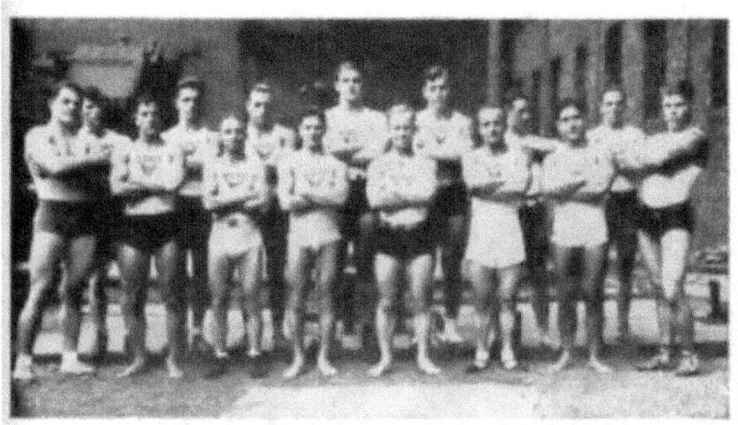

The York team which made lifting history in winning the national team title at the world's fair, Chicago, Ill., 1933. Left to right—Zagurski, Schutt, T. Fiorito, Mitchell, Terlazzo, W. Good, J. Fiorito, Bachtell, Bachtell, W. Good, Levan, Mitchell, Terlazzo, Brown and Miller.

In that year of 1933 the junior national championships were held in the east for the first time. Any men who have not won a junior or senior national title are eligible for that competition. Five members of our team captured titles that year. .So our score for 1933 stood al eight Middle Atlantic titles—all there were—six senior national titles, and five junior national titles—11 national titles in all.

In the next year, members of the York team broke and rebroke American records. That year our lifters scored as follows: in the 112, Frank Tornctta fourth: in the 118, Joe Fiorito third; in the 126, Art Levan first, and Anthony Fiorito fourth; in the 132, Dick Bachtell first, Angelo Taorminc and George Brown third and fourth; in the 148, Bob Mitchell first; Tony Terlazzo dropped out due to a miss on one of the lifts; in the 1C5, Wally Zagurski second; in the 181, Walter Good fourth, and in the heavyweight, Bill Good first.

In the year 1935 in the senior national championships, our team lifted as follows: Joe Fiorito, first in the 118; Art Levan, first in the 126; Darwin Canova, third in the 126;

Dick Bachtell, first in the 132; Angelo Taormine, fifth in the same class; Anthony Terlazzo, first in the 148; Bob Mitchell, second in the 148: John Terpak tied for third in the 148; Walter Good, second in the 165; Wally Zagurski missed a lift in the light-heavyweight class and failed to win the title he had within his grasp; Bill Good was first in the heavyweight division.

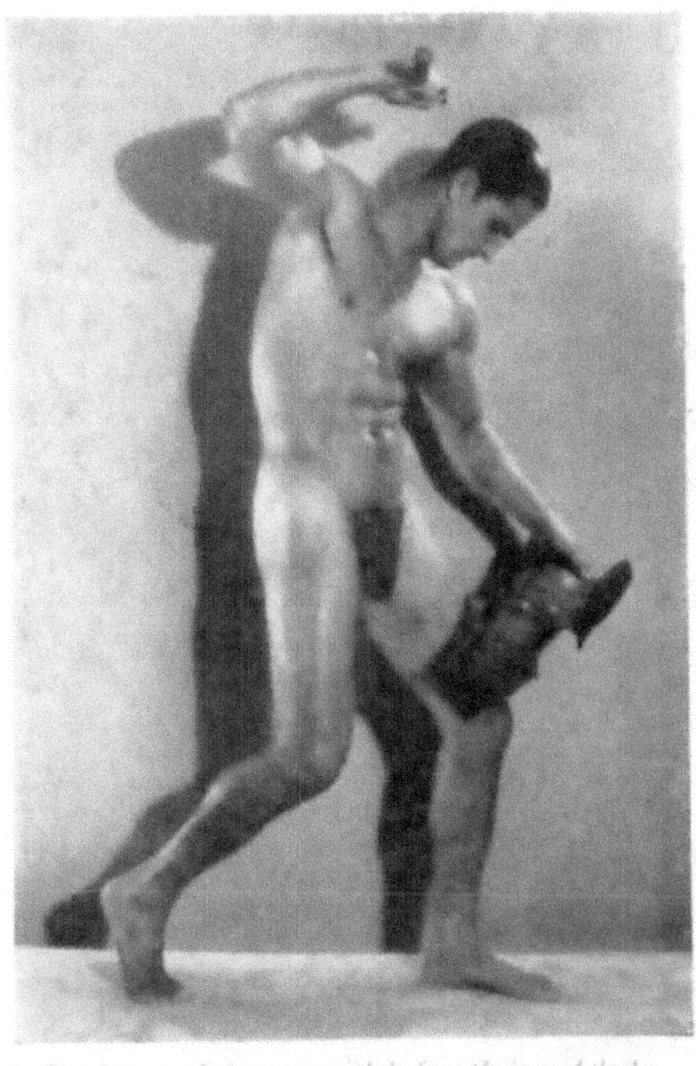

Tony Sansone, who possesses one of the finest physiques of the day.

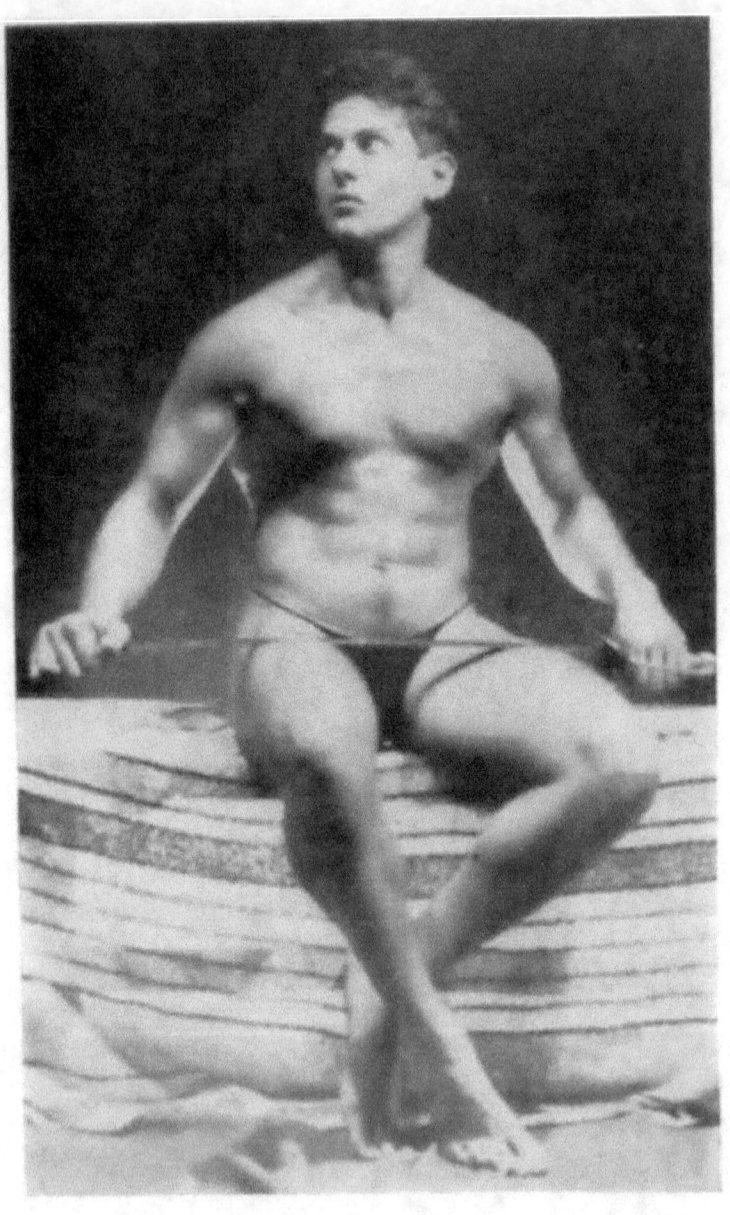

Dave Mayens of Cincinnati, 19 years of age. One of the best built of
the younger generation of lifters.

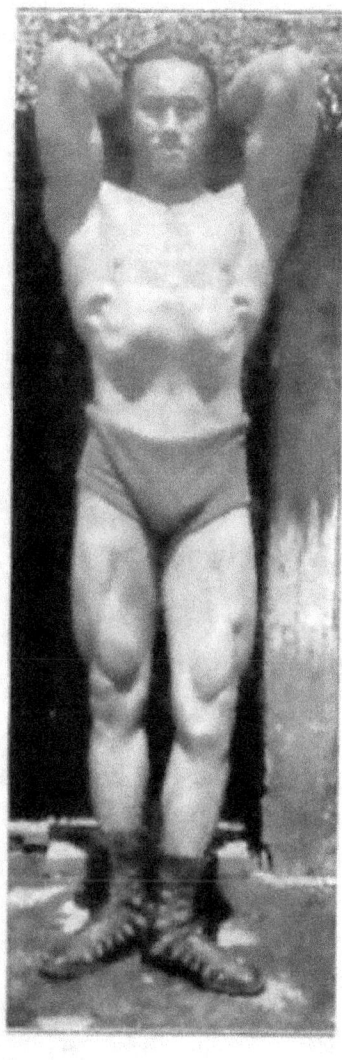

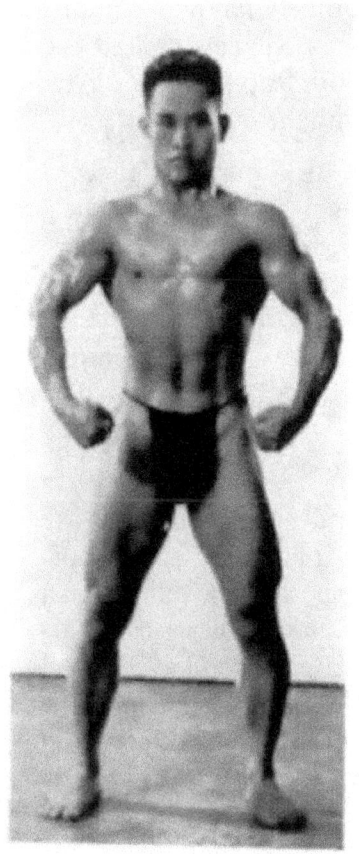

York bar bell men in 32 countries of the world. At left a man from far off China. Below—A powerful little Japanese weight lifter.

In the Olympic year of 1936, York men scored: Joe Fiorito, first in the 118; Darwin Canova, second in the 118; Art

Levan, first in the 126; Tony Terlazzo, first in the 132; Dick Bachtell. third in the 132; Angelo Taormine, sixth in the 132; John Terpak, first in the 148; Bob Mitchell, second in the 148; Pat Napolitana, fifth in the 148; Walter Good, second in the 165; Wally Zagurski, third in the 165; Joe Miller, first in the 181; Gordon Venables tied for second in the 181; Bill Good missed his three presses and did not place; David Mayor, second in the heavyweight and Weldon Bullock, third in the same division. Forty-one points in all were scored by our team.

Of the Olympic team that year, all trained in York. All but one—Stanley Kratkowski - were or are members of the York team, nine of the ten men in all having been affiliated with the York team.

In 1937 our team's record in the nationals was: Joe Fiorito, second in the 126: Dick Bachtell, first in the 132; Tony Fiorito, third in the 126; Tony Terlazzo, first in the 148; Johnny Terpak, first in the 165; Bob Mitchell, second; Wally Zagurski. third in the 181; Dave Mayor, first in the heavyweight and Gord Venables, second. Bill Good who had been a member of our team from the beginning had now withdrawn from our club to go into business with his brother.

And in 1938 the York team again won the national team championship and a good share of the individual titles. This year, 1939, we have many good men; in fact all members of the world's strongest team are members of the club at present. We have no representative in the three smaller classes, having concentrated all our efforts on making men bigger, stronger, better-built and upon the Olympic classes.

At present we have John Terry, senior national 132- pound champion; Dick Bachtell, nine times champion in that class; Lou Schell, a place winner many times in that division; George Brown, who recently won the Interstate Y. M. C. A.

championship in that division; Tony Fiorito; Joe Fiorito, who outgrew the smaller class; and Art Levan, ten times 126-pound national champion, well fortified in that body weight class.

In the 148 we have the national and world's champion in the person of Tony Terlazzo. Although Bob Mitchell has become a professional and is no longer with us we have Eddie Harrison, second only to Terlazzo, former junior national and North American champion, and Val De Genaro who finished third behind these two great lifters last year. In the 165 we have the world's and national champion Terpak, Elmer Farnham, and Elmer Witmer. In the 181 are the world's champion—John Davis the champion of North America, John Grimek, the man who possesses the greatest physique of the day; and in the heavyweight division we have Steve Stanko, the present champion, and Dave Mayor, the former champion, as well as Gord Venables. Bullock has become a professional and is no longer with us.

In addition to the senior national champions mentioned in the preceding paragraphs, the junior national and North American championships our men have won are legion. For instance, Wally Zagurski won five championships in a single year—junior and senior national A.A.U., Middle Atlantic, state and A.C.W.L.A. national. Men whose names have scarcely been mentioned here who have won honors with the York team are Darwin Ganova, champion of North America and junior national champion; Pat Napolitana, former junior national champion; Dave Mayor was junior national champion as was Walter Good: Joe Miller; Bob Mitchell; Harry Thomasillo and many others. Members of the York team have won 54 national titles, senior A.A.U., almost as many North American championships, all of the Middle Atlantic championships year after year, and more than their share of the junior national titles throughout the years.

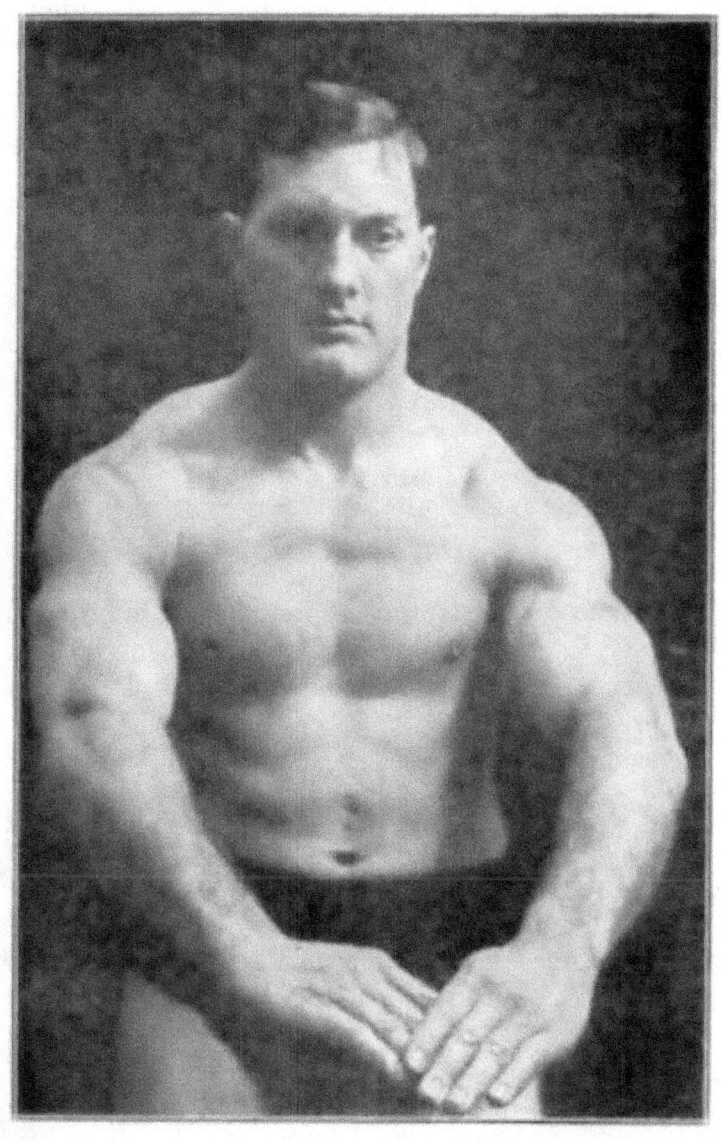

"Wib" Scharzberger, another member of the York team who attained fame for the excellent and powerful physique he developed.

The best records in each division made b\ any lifters in America are as follows:

132-POUND CLASS
Press, 215, Terlazzo, York *
Snatch, 215, Terry, York *
C. & J., 278¾, Terlazzo, York *
Total, 697, Terlazzo, York *

148-POUND CLASS
Press, 255, Terlazzo, York *
Snatch, 248½, Terlazzo, York
C. & J., 335, Terlazzo, York *
Total, 835, Terlazzo, York *

165-POUND CLASS
Press, 260, Terlazzo, York
Snatch, 260, Terpak, York
C. & J., 340, Terlazzo, York *
Total, 845, Terpak, York

181-POUND CLASS
Press, 273½, Davis, York *
Snatch, 275, Davis, York *
C. & J., 353, Davis, York *
Total, 901, Davis, York *

HEAVYWEIGHT CLASS
Press, 322, Davis, York *
Snatch, 317, Davis, York *
C. & J., 382, Stanko, York *
Total, 1020, Stanko, York *

* World's best on record at the time of writing this book.

While it is true that some of these men who are or have been members of the York team were weight lifters before they came to York, they were wise enough to know that their chances of winning weight lifting glory and championships were better if they were here in York where I could personally coach them and help them to reach the heights.

Every man who came to York from some other city came here of his own free will and they stayed because they liked it here. Without exception they showed rapid improvement when they came here, and dropped into lifting mediocrity if they did not continue with the York team. Many lifters quickly catapulted to the top as soon as they became members of our team. There is a tradition that our lifters live up to, and I must admit that they lift harder than they know how to win for myself and the club.

Give me a man who is ambitious, w ho has a burning desire to be a champion and nine times out of ten he will become a champion.

Physical Advantages of Weight Lifting

Uninitiated spectators at a lifting contest may wonder why they do it. They see the magnificent bodies, the splendid muscular development of the enthusiastic strength athletes who enter weight lifting competition and at first thought they believe that these men lift weights to acquire big muscles and the beautiful bodies they possess. For any casual observer will note that weight lifters arc the best-built men in the world. No other sport or athletic pastime creates such powerful, symmetrical, near-perfect development of the human body. Weight lifting brings all the muscles into play and of course it brings all of them to a stage of high development. Just compare the weight lifters whose photos appear in this book and in my largest book, "How to Be Strong, Healthy and Happy," and see how inferior are the men who follow other athletic pastimes, in comparison.

There are men who enter weight lifting competition for the fame it brings them, of course; for the opportunity to win district and national weight lifting titles; to represent their country in the world's championships or the Olympics; the men who have found that weight lifting is the best conditioning sport and practice the weight lifting movements described in this book to improve themselves at some other sport in which they wish to excel; there are some men, greatly in the minority, usually the very young fellows, whose sole desire in practicing weight lifting is to build the most strikingly powerful body, the biggest possible muscles, or the greatest strength. These men are few, although their ambition is a worthy one, for everyone admires a powerful man. Since the beginning of time the strongest men have won the positions of greatest honor, of highest rank, and even in this modern age the strongest, most virile, healthiest men obtain the best positions, win the most attractive or beautiful ladies, gain the best positions and obtain the most from life.

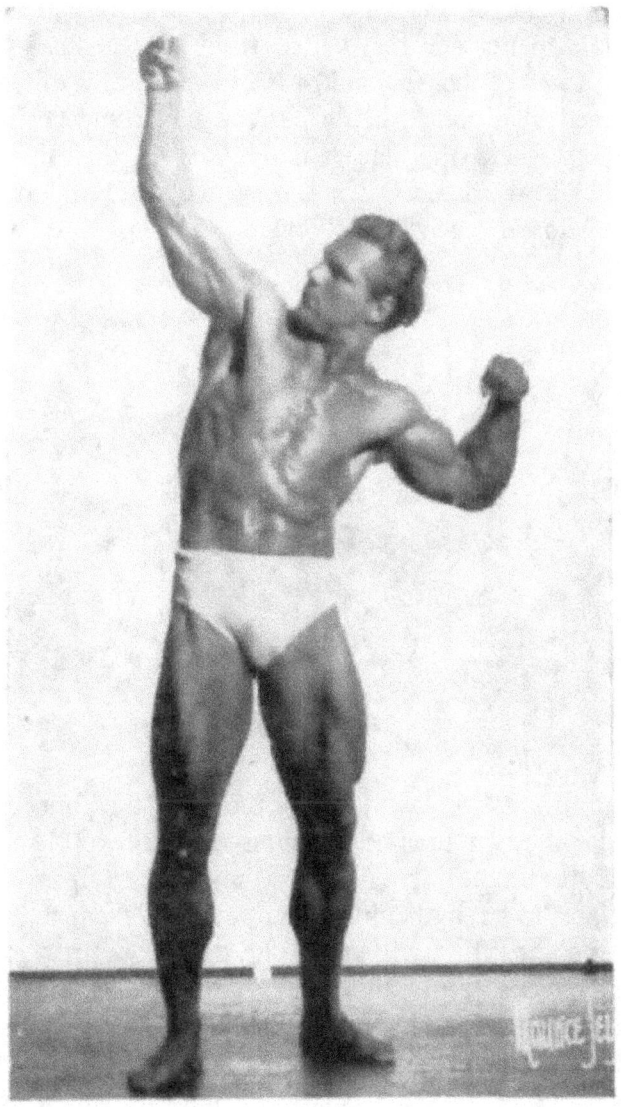

The muscular marvel, John Grimek. The majority believe he has the best physique of the day.

The vast majority of men who enter the field of physical training, as embodied in its advanced state by competitive weight lifting, do so for two reasons: because it makes them look better and feel better. I have stated that weight lifting produces the best-built men in the land. In the best-developed man contests, the perfect man contests, invariably the winners, the place winners and the men to whom the special awards are given—best-developed abdominals, best-developed chest, best-developed arms- are weight lifters.

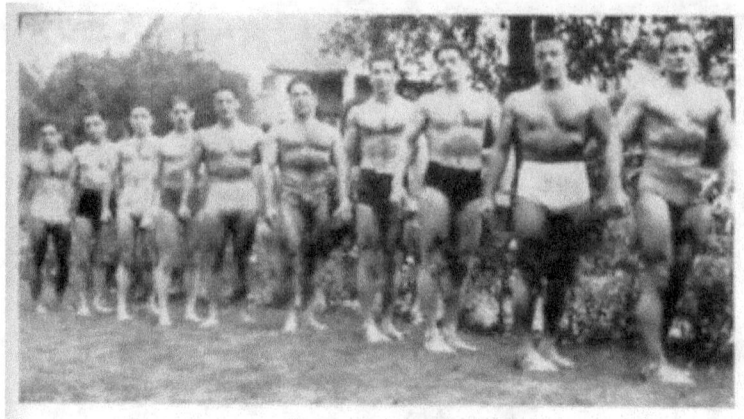

The world's strongest family—the Lapinee Clan. Fifth from the right is Sam Lapinee, internationally famous for the excellency of his physique and the power of his muscles.

Weight lifting brings into play more of the four billion muscular fibres in the body than any form of work, sport or athletic pastime. It strengthens the muscles from even-angle, and in strengthening them develops them to a high state. Weight lifting will fulfill the desire any man should have to possess an admiration-creating, handsome figure. W eight lifting is the best means for the younger, immature man to build his physique. It's the easiest and quickest way too. For unlike some systems of training in which the follower is urged to practice night and morning, seven days a week—fourteen times a week in all—weight lifting brings best results when practiced three or four times weekly, or the system of every other day, three and a half times a week. Only one of these days is it best to make real demands upon the muscles; to urge them to work up to or beyond their best of the past; to make demands upon them which cause them to emerge from their former ruts of inactivity. On the other two training days, more moderate exercises bring best results.

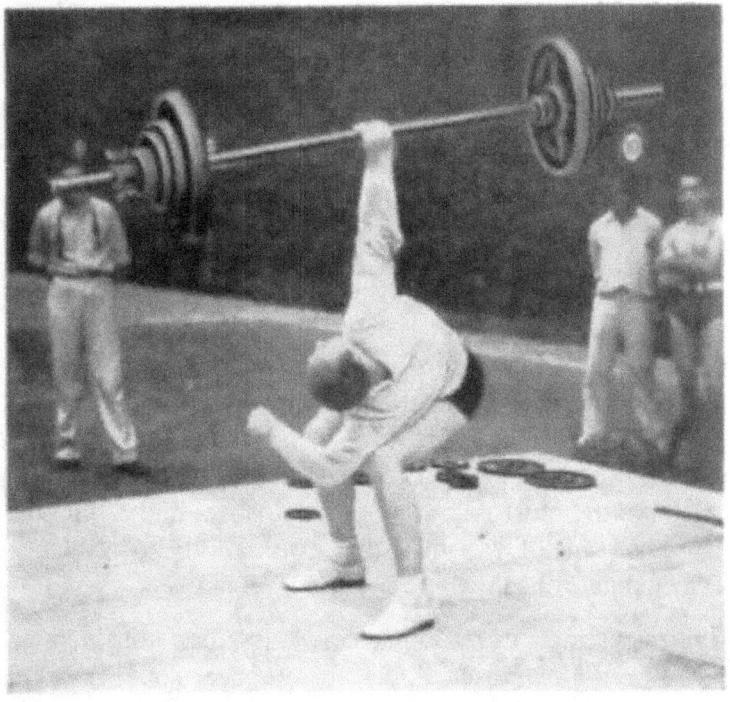

The author at a demonstration of weight lifting in Cuba, early 1939. He is pressing 240 pounds in this photo. Many best presses were a great feat as he is doing to prevent the arm from dipping off the latissimus dorsi while pressing.

For the man who is really ambitious and does not indulge in hard physical work to earn his living, a training system of five days a week will bring best results: for instance, the hardest or limit day Saturday; moderate day Monday; more vigorous day Wednesday; and two other days, Tuesday and Thursday, on which a greater variety of exercises are practiced—those which have been omitted on the real

89

weight lifting days. Rest days, before and after the more vigorous day of training.

This system of training produces more rapid results, although even moderate weight training, when the opportunity offers, will bring splendid results. For weight training is like putting money in the bank. If you save a little now and then, and don't take it out of the bank, your account will grow. Similarly if you train once in a while, it will stamp your physical self with a definite improvement you will experience as long as you live.

Weight training is the easiest, quickest and best method for those older men or women who wish to regain the lost youth, the bodily proportions of youth they let slip away from them through inactivity or wrong living. Mental and physical development and efficiency go hand in hand; both are necessities in building a healthy, happy and successful life. There are such a host of reasons for practicing weight lifting. Improving physical appearance, building those who are underweight, bringing back to normalcy those who are overweight, improving the strength, athletic skill, may seem like the most important effects of weight training, but the best result of weight lifting is its ability to produce a perfect state of health.

And this greatest of reasons receives the least consideration from the non-exerciser. A careful observer could note that champion lifters have pep, energy, bright eyes, super-health; they are light on their feet, constantly filled with boundless energy and endurance. Some may believe that these men were naturally more favored by nature to have reached this highest stage of health and development. But the truth of the matter is, that in the majority of cases, weight lifters were inferior to the average physically in the beginning. A number of cases of outstanding improvement from a very mediocre beginning will be cited later in this chapter.

The majority of men who are the strength champions of today were inferior physically in the beginning and adopted weight training methods to bring their health and their strength up to normal. Many of the champions in the beginning could lift weights which in comparison to their present standards are ridiculously light. Consider at this time the case of Tony Terlazzo, America's most famous weight lifter, Olympic: and world's champion year after year. Although an active, healthy, athletic youth of 19 in the beginning, he could put overhead but 70 pounds. Just recently he pushed the world's record in the two hands clean and jerk in the 148-pound class to an almost unheard-of poundage of 331.

Constant, progressive training through the years brought about this truly amazing improvement. Or another case: Dave Mayor, now a professional heavyweight wrestler, recently national heavyweight amateur lifting champion, weighed 4½ pounds at birth. He weighed 120 when he made his start with bar bell physical training. Four years later he weighed 265 and was America's strongest male. This was solely the result of weight lifting and weight lifting training. Without weight training lie would have been fairly tall and thin, not as strong as the average probably. Or Steve Stanko, America's present strongest man, formerly 120 pounds in weight at his height of nearly six feet. Steve gained over fifty pounds in the first year.

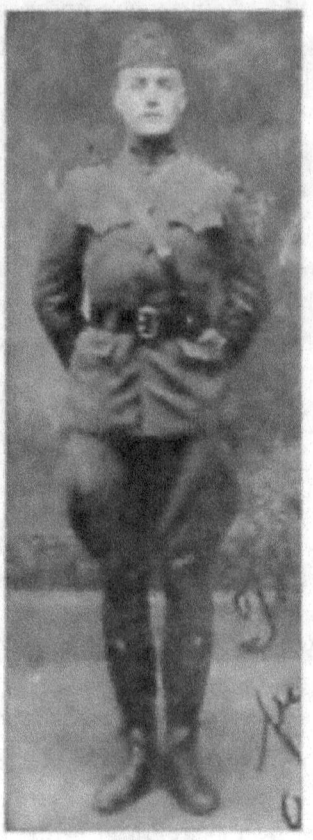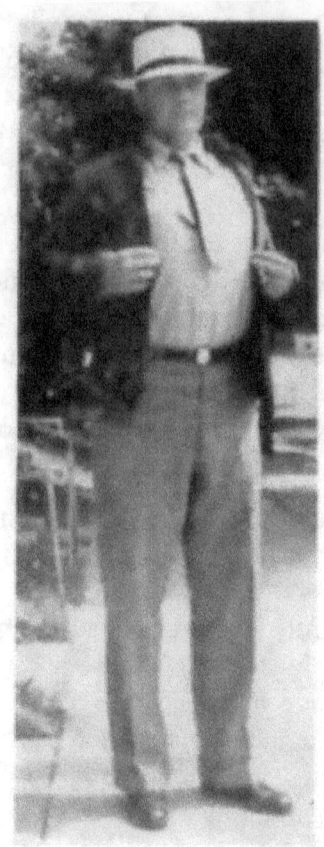

At left—The author in 1919, just after the cessation of hostilities in France. His bodyweight is 150 pounds. A recent picture showing that it is possible to make great improvements in development after the voting age is reached. The coat which fitted loosely in the first photo does not come within a foot of enclosing Bob Hoffman's massive chest.

There are so many cases of men who have overcome severe physical injuries or disease. Roger Eells is perhaps the most famous of these. Although his case has been mentioned on numerous occasions previously, it provides such inspiration to other weaklings that it should be repeated at every opportunity. Roger Eells, now a famous figure in the strength world, the medical world and the field of literature, had the unfortunate experience of being in an advanced stage of tuberculosis just five years ago. He was in such bad shape that he was given three months to live. He sold his business, tried to spend all his money, weighed just 121 pounds. He was still alive at the end of three months and then wondered if there was something he could do about his condition. Exercise was suggested to him, but it seemed impossible at first in his weakened state. He wrote to me, told me his serious condition, wrote that he would take my course of training if I promised him that he would gain twenty pounds. I would not promise. I told him frankly of one or two cases of men who became very strong but had not gained much weight, and I repeated many cases of those who had made phenomenal gains. He- took my course, followed directions and a little over a year later he weighed 160 pounds. As a contrast to his former half-alive, emaciated physique, his face had taken on an athletic, healthy, handsome appearance; his body well-developed, symmetrical proportions. In another year he weighed 180 pounds, had become tremendously strong, and superhealthy. He had been receiving large payments, total disability, from his insurance companies, but upon reading of this phenomenal improvement, the physicians representing the insurance company examined Roger and found him completely cured. The one lung which was completely collapsed, the other about fifty per cent gone, were in perfectly normal condition. They no longer paid him his insurance. This is an authentic case proven by X-rays and reams of scientific data both before and after. Lately Roger Eells put 255 pounds over his head with one arm. He's as handsome and healthy appearing a man as could be found anywhere in the world. Were it not for weight training, undoubtedly he would long ago have become a corpse instead of the fine man he is today.

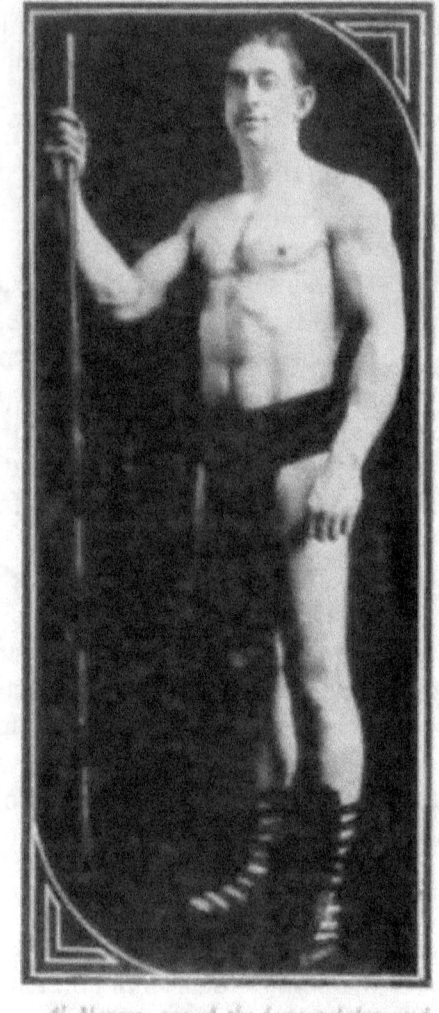

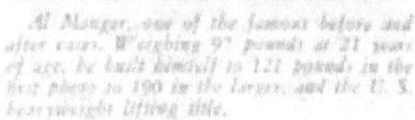

Al Manger, one of the famous before and after cases. Weighing 97 pounds at 21 years of age, he built himself to 121 pounds in the first place to 190 in the larger, and the U. S. heavyweight lifting title.

Another famous case is that of Al Manger of Baltimore. He weighed 97 pounds after the age of twenty-one (unlike the highly advertised 97-pound weakling who claims to have become the world's most perfectly developed man a weight that the story of his life tells us he reached as a boy when he was "healthy and happy as other boys and fond of physical activity"). Manger was mature and thin and undeveloped as a human skeleton. Practicing weight lifting in his bedroom he gained in weight, gained phenomenally in strength and became the United States heavyweight lifting champion, and a member of the 1932 Olympic team.

Art Levan, not so large a man, weighed much less than a hundred pounds when he started. He had a nerve ailment and suffered from periodic attacks of nervous prostration. He became strong through weight training, won ten consecutive senior national A.A.U. weight lifting titles, broke record after record, became the first American to elevate double his weight overhead, and now has built his body to 144 pounds, which Is truly herculean when one considers his small stature. Joe Miller did not have so frail a beginning, but he did increase the size of his chest a full twelve inches in the first year's training, and became one of the world's most powerful men, national weight lifting champion and a member of the Olympic team.

A great many men have overcome some physical defect and reached athletic stardom in spite of it. Johnny Milas, of Akron, minus a lower limb, won his district weight lifting title. Antoine Veiga, due to a childhood injury, has but a thumb, no hand or finger on one hand, and has won his district championship.

A complete story could be written about practically every man who is at present or has been a weight lifting star. Weight lifting miracles are legion. The amazing accounts of their march to physical perfection in spite of a very poor beginning could fill a book many times the size of this one. But I believe the few cases I have offered have given more than a hint of the outstanding physical benefits to be obtained through weight lifting and the training which leads up to proficiency in this fine athletic pastime.

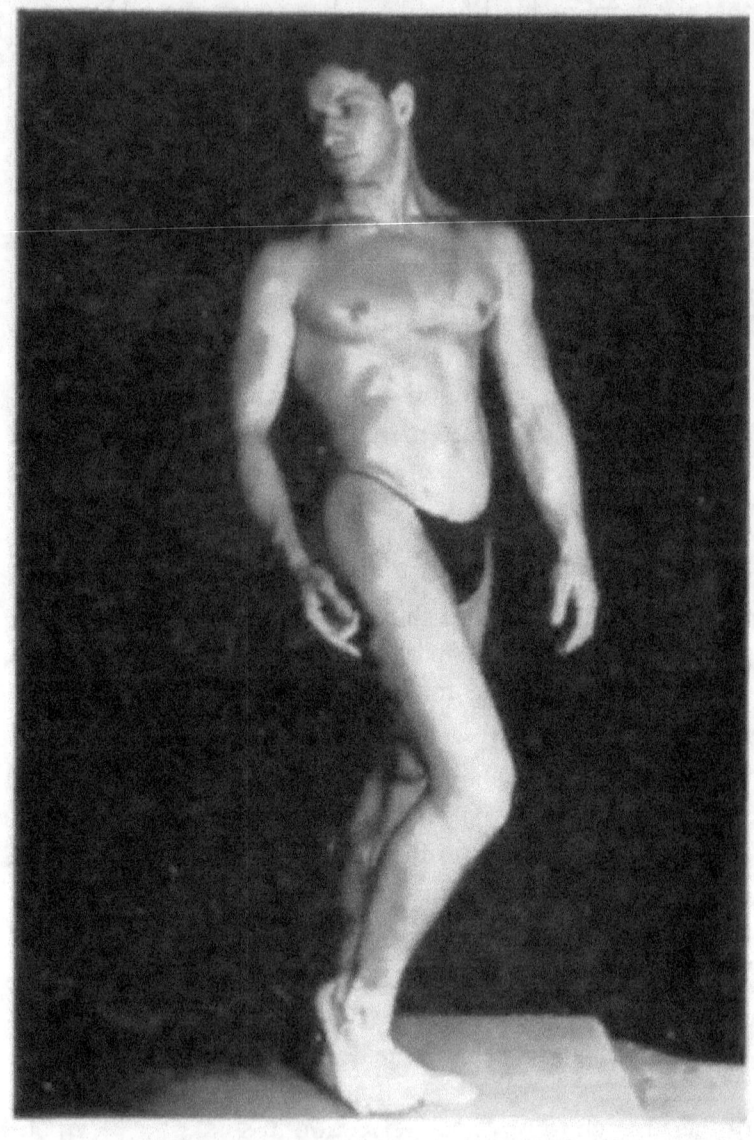

Jack Channing, frequent winner of best physique contests.

One of the first benefits of weight lifting is the beneficial effect it has on improving a man at the branch of athletics he prefers. Weight lifting builds speed, timing, co-ordination, nervous energy, endurance, balance, physical skill and every other desirable physical quality to a great measure. If the athletic star naturally has outstanding ability which makes him an All-American football player, a great wrestler, runner, track and field man, boxer or other athlete, well and good. But if he is below average in the beginning he needs special training to help him reach athletic: heights. And this can best be obtained from special training, such as weight lifting offers.

Nearly every mail I receive brings letters from men who have bettered their time in track events, who have increased their distance in the high or broad jump; who are better pole vaulters, better boxers, better oarsmen, better wrestlers; who have gained a score of pounds and succeeded in making the varsity football team with their added weight and physical ability; who have become home run hitters on their baseball teams, and a great many who have become faster swimmers through their weight-trained muscles.

A few years ago weight training was looked upon with disfavor by the last generation of physical trainers, just a year or two ago, weight lifting was not permitted at the West Point Military Academy, where the future officers who will lead our army units are trained. The weight lifting enthusiasts who obtained appointments there would write to me and state, "What in the world will I do for four years without my weights?" Others "sneaked" back to an abandoned fort on their liberty haul's and practiced with their weights. But recently the West Point authorities have ordered over a half dozen complete weight lifting sets.

Just a few years ago some Y.N.T.G.A.'s were undecided as to whether weight lifting would he beneficial or harmful to the young men who attended their gymnasiums. Some of our star lifters and myself conducted weight lifting clinics at Y. M. C. A. meetings. The "Y" authorities were impressed with the superior type of athletes developed by weight training, and tremendous progress has been made in Y. M. C. A. weight lifting circles. One of these clinics was held at the Pittsburgh Central Y. M. C. A. The meeting was attended by athletic directors from numerous schools of the Pittsburgh district. All went away quite impressed and since that period of only two years ago, many lifting stars have arisen in Pittsburgh. One of their men, a York pupil— Jack Charming——has been acclaimed as one of the best of the younger generation of "perfect men." He has several victories in important perfect man contests to his credit. There was a clinic of sixteen Brooklyn, New York and Long Island Y. M. C. A.'s. They voiced the various objections which had been brought to them in past years. Their objections were overcome when they saw the wonderful athletes I presented, their beautiful physiques, their athletic ability, their strength, their flexibility, and now every one of these Y. M. C. A.'s has large and enthusiastic weight training departments. Brooklyn Central alone has well over 200 regular attendants at their weight training classes, and they produced a man, Joe de Bella, who won the contest to find New York City's best-built man.

Nearly every gymnasium and Y. M. C. A. throughout the nation has become converted to and enthusiastic about weight training. The movement was slow in the beginning, but since our champions have won world-wide acclaim, since Strength and Health magazine has attained its present size and wide circulation, since so many thousands have already received splendid, even incredible results and constantly " tell the world," the weight lifting movement has gone so much faster. In city apartments, on farms, small towns, at widely scattered army posts, in Panama, Hawaii, Alaska, the Philippines, in every state in the Union, nearly every town and city, at schools, universities, ever)'where, weight lifting has made great progress. On the ships of the merchant marine arc found weight lifting enthusiasts. Navy Ships now have weight lifting contests between ships and squadrons as they have long had aquatic events, boxing and wrestling championships.

Truly weight lifting is rapidly reaching the heights. From its little-known beginning a few years ago, from an obscure man here and there who practiced usually alone with a bar bell, there are an estimated more than one million in this country alone who use bar bells, at least ten million who have used them at some stage of their lives.

Dave Aten, who has developed a magnificent torso through weight training.

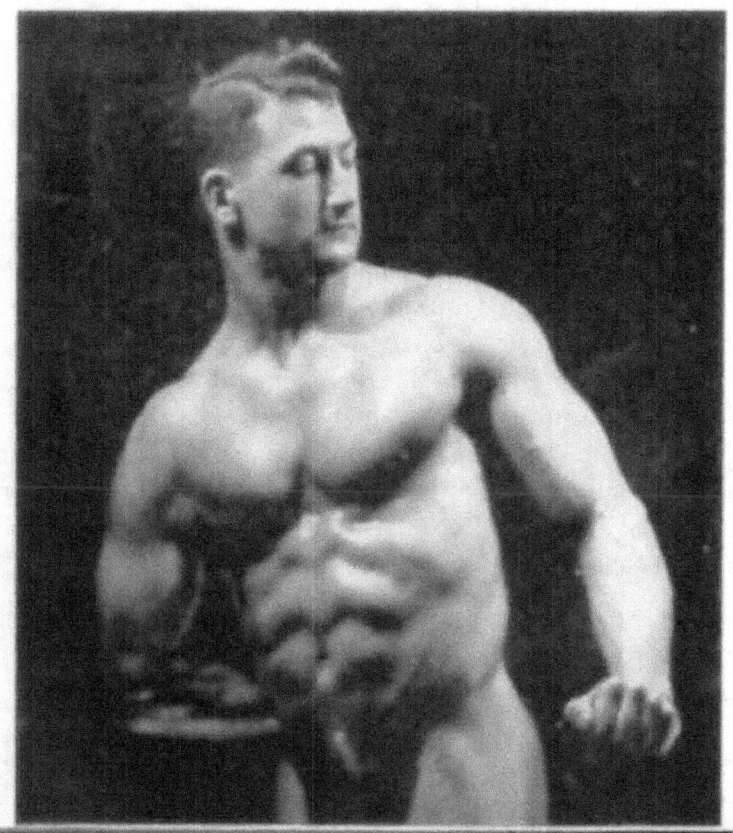

What has caused this great progress in lifting? Chiefly because men who have tried other systems of training with little results have filled their lifelong physical desires improving their strength, appearance and feelings, adding to the length of their lives through weight training—and have constantly told others—more weight lifters, more salesmen for weight lifting. The sport grows by leaps and bounds each year.

What is there about weight lifting, the uninitiated will wonder, that makes it superior to other exercises as a means of physical improvement? I have always said that any exercise is better than no exercise. But most of them do not bring favorable results commensurate with the effort expended. Exercise without apparatus will induce a little perspiration if it is a warm day and the devotee of that form of exercise is sufficiently enthusiastic. It will stir up the action of the blood just a little, cause a bit faster breathing. But soon the muscles become accustomed to the effort required of them and after the first few days or weeks, 110 further gains are made. It Is nature's plan to try to fulfill the demands made of the muscles. If you wave the arms around you become just strong enough to wave the arms around. If you bend from side to side or even touch the toes, you become just strong enough to perform those movements. Even the more vigorous without apparatus movements of chinning and floor dipping arc not progressive; too hard for a big man or woman, too easy to bring maximum results for a light man.

But in weight lifting we have a form of exercise that is really progressive. The frailest man or woman can select exactly the poundage that suits them best in every exercise. Straining is not recommended in weight exercising; rather, moderate, constantly progressive training. The bar with one of the exercise sets weighs only five pounds. If the beginner is small, sickly or frail the start can be made with just five pounds. Then movements up to ten are practiced. It is recommended that the weight one can comfortably handle be employed. There is a quick response to the exercises and the weights are increased in jumps as small as $1^1/_4$ pounds. Gradually over a period of time, strength, energy and endurance increase and heavier poundages can be utilized. While the average beginner may use as little as thirty-five pounds in the two hands curl and fifty in the two hands press, some of I he advanced bar bell men refuse in any training period to employ less than two hundred in pressing, three hundred in deep knee bending, four hundred in dead weight lifting, and one hundred and twenty- five pounds in two arm curling. Heavier weights bring more rapid results with a smaller expenditure of time and effort. These seem like great poundages to the beginner. But I can assure you that most of the present strength stars could handle no more than the light poundages mentioned in the beginning. Constant training brought them their strength and development so gradually that it was hardly noticeable, until one day they began to attract favorable attention and the enthusiastic remarks of their friends. Where does all this increased strength, development and better internal feeling come from, you will wonder?

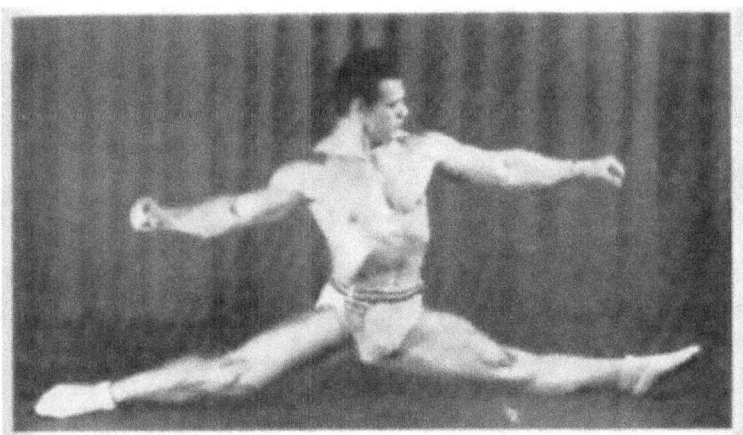

Weight lifting champion John Grimek, probably the most muscular man in America at present, demonstrating the flexibility of his muscles. Advanced bar bell men are the most flexible of men and can perform feats which real those of a contortionist.

I could go on indefinitely offering more reasons why weight lifting is beneficial for men and women of all ages. It's especially fine for those at the period of puberty, of most rapid growth. Younger brothers who take up weight training invariably grow larger and stronger than their father or older brothers. A few weeks of weight training will help you really appreciate it.

The Best System of Physical Training

Weight lifting builds the muscles. That's evident. They can be seen so easily by a visitor to any weight lifting contest or strength and health display. But what we can't see is the great improvement, the great strengthening of every internal process, of every organ and gland, for the muscles could not be improved without this beneficial effect in the internal processes. Making demands on the muscles causes the internal organs to work more intensively and more efficiently. This in turn aids the muscles in their gains of size, shapeliness and strength. More weight can be handled, more weight can be lifted; there is more improvement in the internal processes, more improvement in the muscles. The organs and muscles inside work in unison with the outer muscles of the body.

The chief benefit of weight lifting is this improvement of the inside of the body. We can be neither strong nor healthy unless we have a powerful, proper functioning set of internal machinery. The active muscles must be fed, nourished and provided with fuel and power by our internal organs. Through progressive weight training the organs and glands are taught to function at a high degree of efficiency. When these organs are strengthened, their operation improved, a reserve of vital energy is produced. The resulting strengthening of the organs brings a greater prospect of long life and greatly reduces the possibility of contracting a disease which may shorten the life or end it suddenly and prematurely. Pep, energy, vitality, endurance, wind, courage, determination, ambition, are all products of internal strength. A pure blood stream, strong respiratory and circulatory processes and strong nerves make the muscles powerful and more enduring.

Life Ls lengthened when the internal organs and glands are strengthened because people die when one or more of the internal organs fail to function. Anything that is done to improve their operation, strengthen them, increase their length of efficient usefulness, adds to the length of the life of the person who owns and depends upon these organs. Statistics prove that forty per cent of the people who leave this world make their too often premature exit through heart ailments of various sorts. A large percentage of deaths are caused by kidney diseases. A complication of diseases takes many others to the great beyond.

We may complain at times about the world and its policies, but life is sweet and few of us want to leave the world. We'd like to remain here as many years as possible. To do this, and to fully enjoy those years while we are here, we need strong hearts, powerful lungs, good kidneys, capable livers, and a digestive and eliminative system that performs its work well. Our entire future lives depend on the capabilities of the stomach and other allied organs—the intestines, organs of elimination, ff just one of these functions fails to do its work, sickness or death, too often a painful form of death, is the result.

What's all this got to do with weight lifting you may be wondering. A great deal, I can assure you. You depend on these organs. Your life depends on them. In turn they depend on you, upon the care you give them. You are in partnership with them, must pull together with them if you want to live long and fully. The organs can't tell you what is wrong with them, but they can cause you plenty of pain when they don't feel right. They can't obtain their own food, their own exercise, so you, their owner, must provide the nourishment and the stimulation.

You can feed them by supplying their needs. Eating good foods at meal times only. Good lean meat, beef, mutton, chicken or fish are best. Plenty of body building vegetables—those of a leafy nature fruits, too, serve as bodily cleansers and supply the vitamins and minerals the body requires.

You must see that the body obtains sufficient rest and relaxation and after that, exercise, stimulation of these organs, is the all-important need. Since the organs need exercise, there is only one way to exercise them. That is to exercise the muscles. It has been proven that light exercises provide little benefit for the outer muscles, less for the inner works. Greater demands must be made upon the muscles to improve them and greater effort is then required of the internal works, with increasing benefit to them.

A man with weak muscles makes his beginning in weight training with moderate resistance and few repetitions. More and more weight is handled as the muscles gradually respond to the progressive resistance. The muscles are trained, coaxed along, and as they increase in size, strength and efficiency, their partners, the organs, are improved in similar manner. As it's the work of the organs to feed, provide fuel and to drive the muscles, better operating and stronger muscles are built, really as a result of having built better functioning and stronger organs and glands. We must constantly remember that it is the organs which drive the muscles which in turn push, carry, lift or Dull as directed by the mind.

You can't see what goes on inside of you, but die improvement I am describing takes place just the same. If you start to run a little each day, or to perform so many movements with bar bells or dumbells, after a short period of (raining you will find yourself able to run a little farther, to perform a few more repetitions or to handle more weight for these repetitions. This condition has come about through the better operating organs and glands. Circulation has been speeded up and improved, it carries away the worn or broken-down tissue and replaces it with additional fresh building material with ever-increasing speed as greater demands are made. Respiration improves, for weight training causes faster breathing, and this improves the blood stream, impregnates it with life-giving oxygen which unites with the glycogen, providing combustion, and in turn power in the muscles. Profuse perspiration is the natural result of exercise and this carries a great deal of the bodih waste to the outside through the pores. The kidneys have less work to do and arc able to do more when called upon. Weight training rubs, massages, exercises the internal organs as the outer muscles are exercised. This helps digestion and elimination. Demands have been made upon the body, so assimilation is bettered. As the body requires fuel and power to perform the exercises, the material it needs is drawn from the body, hastening digestion, improving assimilation and metabolism.

Every action of our daily lives causes some stimulation of the internal organs. If you walk upstairs, or run for the train, you'll notice that your heart pumps harder and that you breathe faster and more fully. And the more you move, the more you work, the more exercise your internal works receive. Just as the muscles strengthen with this work, the organs strengthen too. As the muscles arc gradually trained to push harder, to lift more weight, this gradual improvement comes about because the organs are improving too.

Thus the strongest men have the strongest organs. The strongest men have the strongest hearts, for the heart is a muscle which is strengthened with use, especially when its tissues are fed with the proper food elements. The increased breathing greatly strengthens the lungs. The best kidneys, and liver, a powerful stomach, good digestion, and the strongest, most prolific glands have strength in their respective parts in direct proportion to the strength of the outer muscles. All of which results in longer life, a fuller life, more sexual power for the strong man. Strong men, star weight lifters, have amazing appetites and the finest operating internal works that could be had. To mention my own case for instance: I haven't had a headache or a sick stomach for thirty years—not since I was a child and learned how and what to eat. I, like other weight lifters, am never bothered by the host of minor ailments such as belching, gas, heartburn, pimples or boils, no infection—injuries heal quickly—or other minor or major eliminative and digestive complaints. The organs of the star weight lifter synchronize and operate more efficiently, when properly treated and properly exercised, than do the parts of the finest and most intricate man-made machine. Gradually progressive resistance, constantly increasing the strength of muscles by handling ever heavier weights, is the way to superorganic action which in turn results in a longer, fuller, happier life.

Few men indeed would exercise just to get big muscles on the outside of the body, were it not for the greatly improved appearance, the superior feelings, the happier and longer life, the development of the muscles will produce.

You may be wondering why, if all the benefits I am describing as a result of weight training are true, they cannot be obtained from work or other forms of exercise.

Ladies will say that they get plenty of exercise caring for their children and doing their housework. That's work, not exercise. It's just what hundreds of millions of women are doing throughout the world, yet they turn out in many cases to be shapeless, unhealthy, sad-looking caricatures of what real women should be. Men in turn say that they obtain plenty of exercise in doing their daily work, in earning their living. Yet few men are in the condition that nature intended them to be. For work is not exercise. Work is exhausting, as arc most forms of exercise. They demand far more of the body than they produce in the way of beneficial effects. You must have noticed that few of the men who do the world's work, the laborers, arc either well developed, healthy, or nice appearing. Through the work that they have done, their strength, power and energy have flown out of the body. It is a vital loss, something gone from the body, which must be replaced in some manner. And the best way to replace it is through weight lifting, right eating and good sound sleep in sufficient quantities to thoroughly rest the body.

Weight lifting as we scientifically teach it brings power back into the body. It recharges your inner organs and cells. For weight lifting produces so much more than it demands. If you can picture for a minute a poorly operating generator in a car, which does not produce enough current to replace that used in the operation of the car—the spark plugs, horn, starter, lights, radio—gradually permitting the battery to become weaker until it must be replaced or recharged, and then think of a powerful generator producing more than enough current for all the needs of the car, you will have in the former case a condition similar to the result of work and in the latter case a similarity to the favorable results of weight lifting exercises.

Work is work, and exercise is relaxation—pleasure, for most persons -and even if you loathed it, abhorred it, disliked and hated it it would still bring favorable results, although the greatest benefits are obtained if you enjoy your exercise and obtain pleasure from it. For the mental driving that is necessary at work, in performing some task that is distasteful, forms lactic acid in the working muscle and greater or lesser fatigue in direct proportion to the effort you force yourself to put forth.

A muscular fuel, glycogen, is brought from the bodily storehouse while the muscle is working. Oxygen is required for combustion with this energy-creating substance. And right here is where the trouble develops through work; why it makes you tired. The respiration is not stimulated, the circulation is not amplified, as it is with weight lifting, so the blood ran not carry enough oxygen to burn sufficient glycogen to keep the muscles working efficiently. An oxygen debt is piled up, which requires considerable time to recuperate from.

Weight lifting or heavy weight training increases the tempo of the respiration; it speeds up the circulation. Thus, a great deal more oxygen than is required to perform the particular movement being practiced is brought to the working muscles. This action revitalizes the tired body, or peps up one in the toils of simple inertia. The exhausted cells of the physical organism arc recharged. Work or light exercise which does not cause this increased respiration and circulation wears down your cellular structure. Scientific-weight training builds it up. There's a big difference between light exercise or work, and heavy exercise. Any man who has advanced to the point in weight training where he can handle truly heavy poundages will enjoy a thrilling feeling of exhilaration, of energy at the completion of his training period, an indescribable feeling of pep and well-being. This comes as the result of building up more than the body requires, just like the well-charged battery can whirl the motor of the car in starting, and have more than enough to spare for all the work it is designed to do.

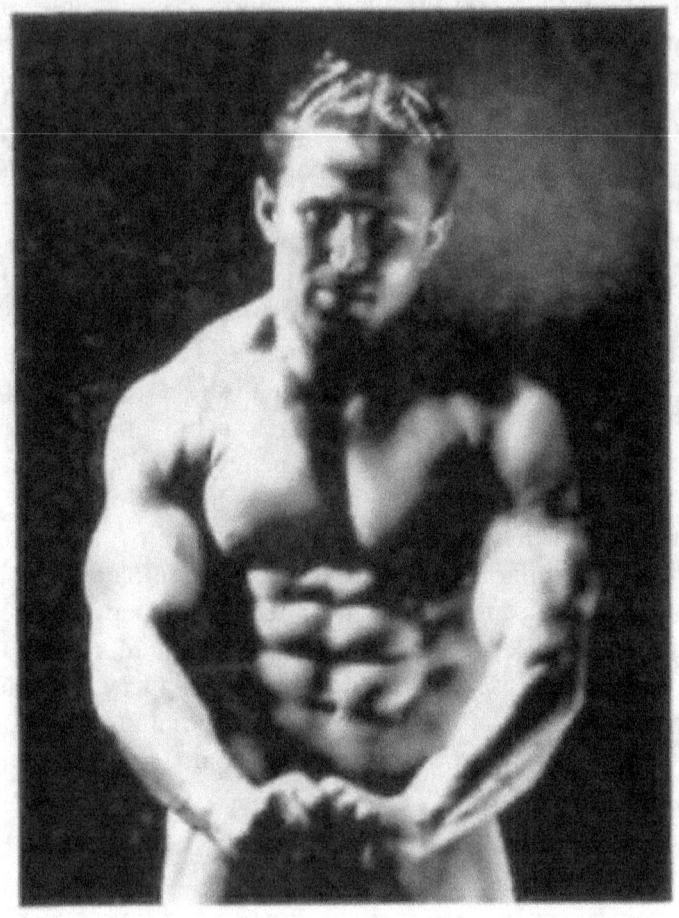

Tony Petroline of Chicago, formerly a fat man of nearly two hundred pounds. Weight training and lifting built for him this splendidly proportioned 165-pound physique.

If work or light exercise were all that was required to make people well and strong, nearly every man would he a superman—well, strong and healthy. But it's evident that work alone is not the answer, for hard-working men are subject to every ill that comes along. Hard work brings bent, ugly, malformed, misshapen, fat or obese, out-of-shape bodies. Scientific exercise not only eliminates this condition in men or women of any age, but builds up superhealth besides.

There are over 520 muscles in the body. So there is not a single line of work or athletics with the exception of weight training that will properly develop all of these muscles. The ambitious weight lifter not only practices a wide variety of lifts, but exercises muscles in groups to improve them in strength, appearance and physical ability. These muscles vary in strength from the terrifically powerful extensors of the lower limbs, muscles which can press out many hundreds of pounds, to the muscles of the deltoids which permit the holding out of little more than fifty- pounds even by those men who are quite strong. Hundreds of pounds are required to fully develop some of the muscles; only ten pounds by others. It's evident that specialized training with graded resistance, a system of training possible only with bar bells and dumbells, is required to bring out the ultimate in strength, health and development.

Weight training brings greater physical benefit than any form of work or exercise. The physical results obtained are the main reason why weight lifting has grown by such leaps and bounds, why its devotees include the best built and strongest men in the land. I'll take up the remainder of this chapter with a partial list of reasons why weight lifting is beneficial; why it is a sport which should be practiced by every man and woman of every age, from the teens to near the Biblical prophecy of threescore and ten: why every school, home and organization should influence its members to practice weight training—moderately for those who wish only to keep fit, more intensively for those who wish to become supermen and women. For weight lifting benefits in direct proportion to the amount of effort put forth. More work, greater results and less exercise time arc required in this latter case.

1.   Weight lifting speeds up the circulation, keeps the blood coursing through the body. Sluggish circulation is the cause of much pain and discomfort. In normal persons there is only one-sixth as much blood in circulation below the ankles as above. No wonder your feet often hurt and are cold. Better circulation is a principal result of heavy exercise.

2.   Scientific weight training improves the function of all the internal organs; it builds their strength. It makes all the organs and glands more active. It makes it possible for all organs and glands to perform their functions more healthfully and normally.

3.   Proper elimination of waste from the body is one of the chief results of weight training. Leading medical men and physical directors of today believe that at least ninety per cent of all diseases arc the result of internal filth, of faulty and inadequate elimination. If you know anyone who is constipated, taking laxatives, they need proper exercise.

4.   Lactic acid and other fatigue poisons are removed through weight training.

5.   Exercise creates demands upon the body. It breaks down tissue and with the help of improved circulation and proper eating it builds new, stronger and healthier cells.

6.   " Activity is life," '.' stagnation is death," " in life there is movement "—are all well-known truisms. And weight lifting exercises, bringing healthful activity to every organ, gland and cell of the body, keep the entire body and mind

radiantly alive and with a feeling of pep, energy and well-being that makes one so buoyant and alive they feel like jumping, running or dancing.

7.   Weight lifting provides diversion, new interest, stimulates circulation, purifies the blood that feeds the

mind as well as other parts of the body, thus making the mind clear, alert and sparkling. Students who practice weight training are apt to be leaders in their classes, receive the highest grades in their studies and graduate with honors.

8.	Weight training builds co-ordination, balance, control of all the muscles; it builds speed, judgment of time, space and distance. It makes the entire body more responsive to the will, and it teaches the body to do the right thing in time of danger even before it is directed by the mind. Thus an accident, perhaps one that would be fatal, is so often avoided and the span of life lengthened. Many men are alive today because their muscles were trained, did the right thing at the right time, thus saving their lives.

9.	Weight lifting is the best insurance against disease or sickness. It builds a fund of resistance, of healthy blood, both white and red corpuscles, which can attack and over-come any disease germs which come in contact with the body. Strong men are seldom sick or ailing.

10. Weight lifting builds confidence, for there is no road to supreme confidence as sure as the knowledge of one's physical and mental ability. It cultivates power of will, produces complete mastery of your physical and mental self, promotes personal efficiency and all desirable mental characteristics.

11. Weight lifting improves the efficiency of every part of the body. It helps you be happier. It provides pleasurable interest and diversion to your exercise. There's a thrill in outlifting your friends or teammates, in bettering your own lifetime records. It helps you sleep sounder and faster, so that you have more time for work or pleasure. It makes it possible for you to earn more.

12.	Weight lifting makes it possible for you to live more. As the glands adjacent to the working musc.lcs arc improved through weight lifting exercises, you are able to love more.

13.   Although we do not recommend irregularities of living or dissipation, if you insist on going to a party and indulging in harmful practices, which we diagnose as leaks, abuses (perhaps minor ones) against the body, you will not experience the morning after headaches, bad taste and lack of pep you would if you did not exercise. The man who lifts weights has a much more healthy, active body, organs that can throw off or overcome the products of bad food, liquor, too much smoking and other excesses.

14.   Exercise is the best insurance known. The moderate time that weight lifting exercises require will pay you a thousand times in dividends of physical benefits.

15.   Weight lifting is a pleasure. It provides a lifelong hobby, an additional interest in life. It will make many friends for you—good, wholesome fellows. For those who reach the heights in lifting, it has provided world-wide travel, international acclaim. But even if you are not interested in competitive weight lifting it will prove to be the greatest force for physical and mental benefit in your entire life.

16.   Weight lifting has been responsible for the development of the best built men past and present. The winners and place winners of best physique contests are invariably weight trained men. Weight lifting will quickly build two or three times the strength of the average man and a striking appearing, admiration creating figure.

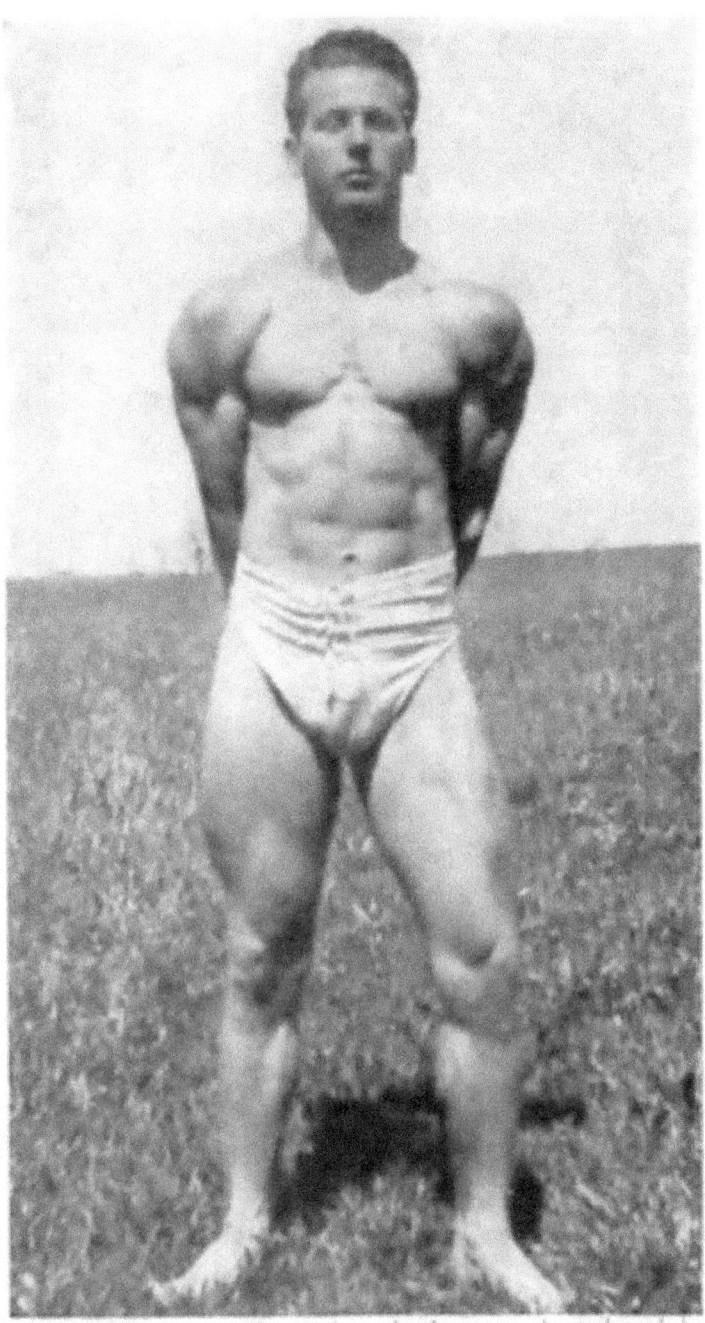

Dick Zimmerman, another York youth who rose to fame through his hard bell built muscles. Dick and his younger brother Joe have attained great fame as professional performers.

Fundamental Lifts

ABDOMINAL RAISE

Official Definition

Lift No. 1—Lie upon the floor with the back of the neck against the center of the bar bell. Grasp the bar bell with both hands and from that position raise to a sitting position. It is permissible to place the feet under some heavy object, and the heels must be kept together, the legs held straight throughout the lift, the bar against the back of the neck or shoulders. At the completion of the lift, the body is at right angles to the legs. It is not permissible to use a dumbell in performing this lift.

Method of Performance

Load the bar bell to the desired weight. Lie Hat upon the floor, placing the body so that the neck is against the middle of the bar. Grasp the bar with the hands a little less than shoulder width apart. It is permissible to hold the feet down and this is best done by thrusting them under another loaded bar bell. The feet must be held firmly under the bar, the heels kept together, the legs held straight throughout, and then the body is raised until it reaches the position at right angles to the legs, when the count of two is taken.

Causes for Disqualification are: the bending of the legs, separating the heels throughout the lift, the failure to raise the upper body to the upright position, the removal of the bell from the shoulders during the progress of the lift, of the use of a bar bell with plates larger than ten inches.

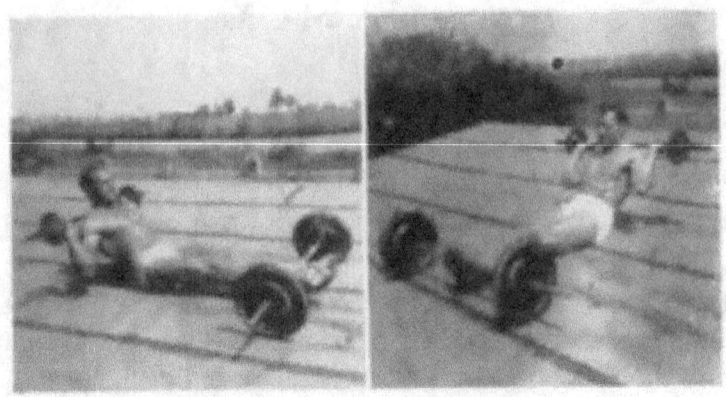

Abdominal raise. Posed by Elmer Farnham and John Grimek.

PULL OVER AT ARM'S LENGTH

Official Definition

LIFT NO. 2.—Lie upon the floor with the arms extruded to their full length bark of head. From this position, keeping the arms straight throughout, the bur is raised until it is at right angles to the body. While the lift is in progress the heels must be kepi together, the legs perfectly straight and the bullocks in contact with the floor. The use of a dumbell in this lift is not allowed.

Method of Performance

Assume the supine position with back to floor, and a bar bell within reach back of head. Grasp the bar with the hands approximately shoulder width apart and an equal distance from the center of the bar. The object of the lift is to raise the bell in a semicircular movement, keeping the arms straight throughout, until it is directly over the hair of the lifter.

It is very important that the hands lie the proper distance from the center of the bar. If a York liar bell is employed, placing the hands at the inside of the knurling is the best position. The heels must be kept together throughout the lift, the legs straight and the buttocks against the floor. When the bell is directly above the body the count should be taken.

This lift is a good exercise, one which should be normally practised with a moderate weight which can be easily and properly handled. As a lift or strength feat of course the object is to handle the greatest weight which can be properly lifted within the interpretation of the rules.

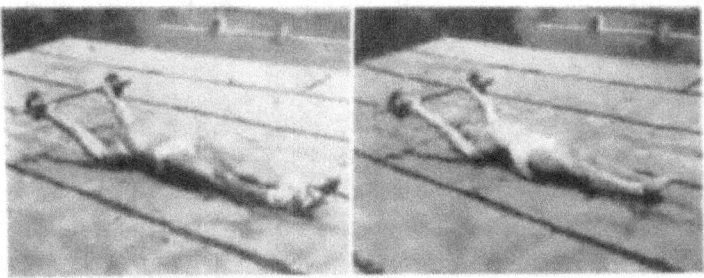

Pull over at arm's length. Posed by Elmer Farnham and John Grimek.

TWO HANDS DEAD WEIGHT LIFT

Official Definition

LIFT NO. 3.—The bar bell must be lifted from the floor until the lifter is erect with straight back. Il is optional whether the heels be kept together or approximately shoulder width apart. But the legs must be straight, the back straight and the shoulders back at the completion of the lift. The lifter may hold the bar as he likes and the bar can touch the thighs in the progress of the lift.

Method of Performance

Stand with the feet well under the bell in the position that practice has shown you to be most comfortable and the one in which you can exert the greatest force. In England it Is a rule that the heels must be together, but in this country many of the best dead weight lifters stand with the feet at least shoulder width apart. The hands are usually held with

119

the palms facing each other. In the French style it is necessary that the knuckles be held front, as in pulling bell to chest, but any position of the hands is permissible. Some of the best lifters use a rather wide grip, much more than shoulder width apart, others with the hands at just a bit more than shoulder width. Assume the position that practice teaches you to be best in your particular case.

The start in the dead weight lift is the same as that of any of the quick lifts such as two hands snatch or two hands clean—the buttocks lowered, the back flat and curved in slightly, the arms hanging straight and loosely. When power is applied, the head is raised, the knees are bent slightly outward and there is an endeavor to raise the shoulders. Straighten the back and the legs almost simultaneously, until at the completion of the lift the shoulders arc back, the head erect and the back straight. When that position is assumed the count is taken.

Causes for Disqualification are: Legs not straight; trunk not erect; the shoulders not back at the completion of the lift.

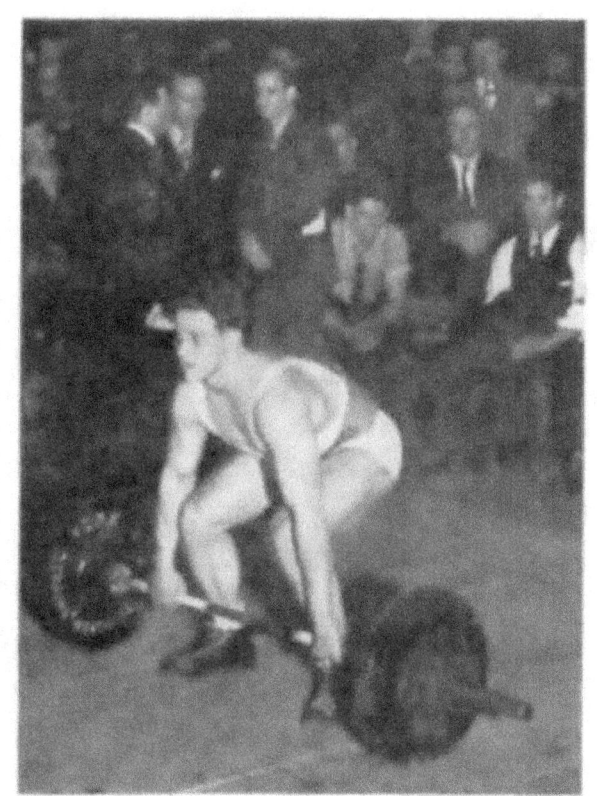

Louis Abele, one of America's greatest heavyweight lifters, nineteen years of age in this photo. His record on the clean and jerk is 330 pounds. This position is ideal for the start of the dead lift, two hands snatch, two hands clean or for any form of cleaning the weight to the shoulders.

STIFF LEGGED DEAD WEIGHT LIFT

Official Definition

Lift No. 4.—This lift is performed in similar style to the regular two hands dead weight lift except that the knees must be locked and the heels kept together throughout the lift.

Method of Performance

Stand with the feet well under the bar bell, heels together, knees straight. Bending from the back entirely grasp the bar with the palm of one hand to the front, the other to the rear. The hands should be spaced the distance apart that practice has found to be best for you. Grip the bar tightly, raise the shoulders and straighten the back simultaneously. This is a lift which requires flexibility of the back, and great power in that region. The average performer can not lift as much weight in this style as with the bent knee, back flat method. But it is a great developing exercise. Complete the lift by standing with the head erect, the shoulders back and the back straight.

Causes for Disqualification are: Bending the legs during the progress of the lift; and at the completion of the lift the failure to have back straight, head erect, and shoulders bark.

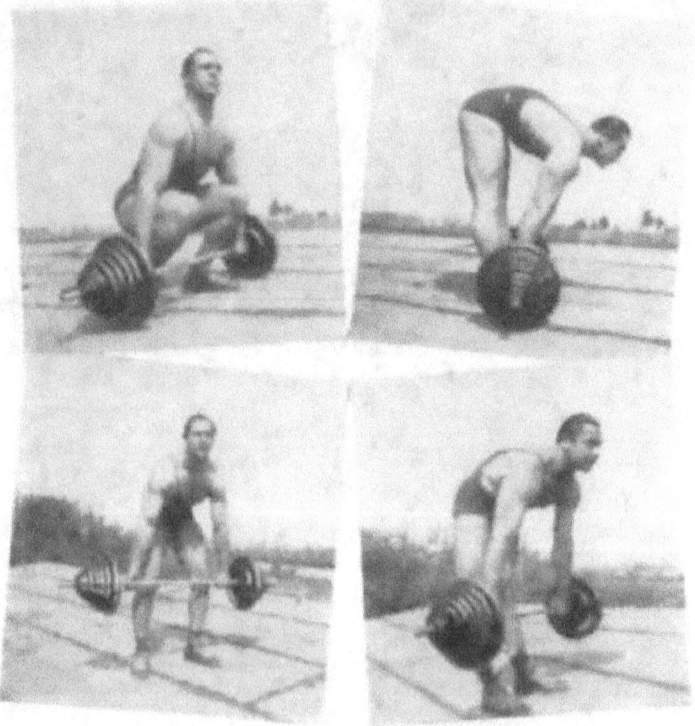

The stiff legged dead weight lift, starting position and half way through the lift. The regular two hands dead weight lift, starting position and part way up with the weight. Posed by Steve Stanko.

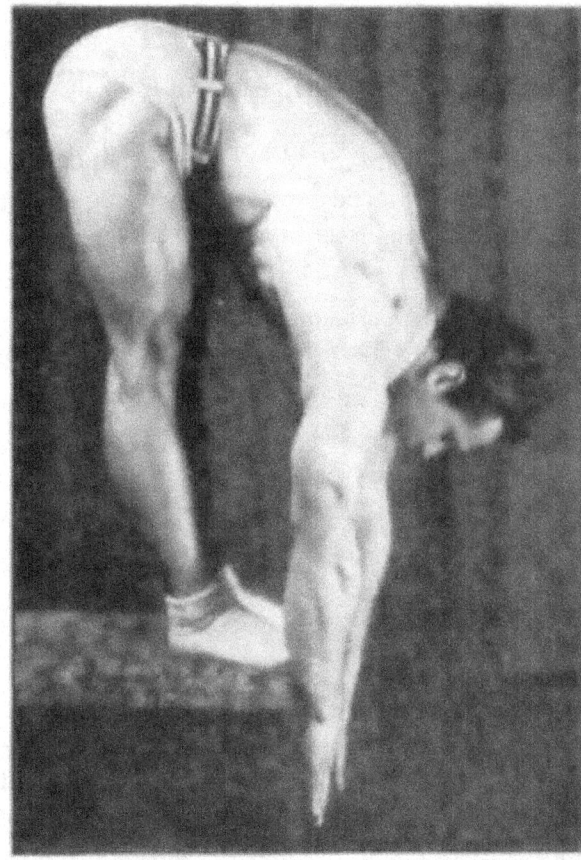

LEFT HAND DEAD WEIGHT LIFT

Official Definition

LIFT NO. 5.—At the beginning 0/ the lift the bar bell may lie either at right angles to or parallel to the front of the lifter. From that position it must be lifted from the floor, at least to the height of the lifter's knees. The legs must be straight and knees locked at the completion of the lift. The feet remain astride throughout the lift.

Before making the lift, locate the exact center of the bell. This is easily found by raising the bar with the lifting hand in the proper position, the other hand beneath it. As you prepare to lift, stand over the weight with the feet about shoulder width apart and the heels equidistant from the bar. Keep the back flat, bend the knees outward, and grasp the bar at the point you previously found to be the exact center. The non-lifting hand is placed upon the corresponding thigh with the thumb and fingers turned in.

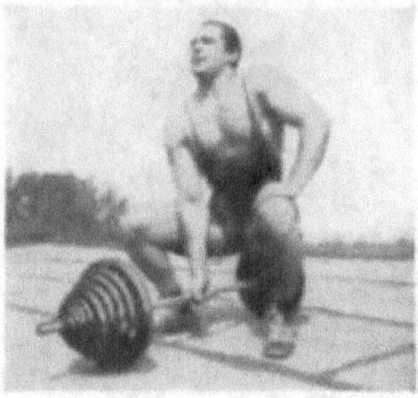

Start of the one hand dead weight lift.

The amount of weight which can be lifted in this style depends upon the gripping power. It is permissible to cm-ploy a hook grip. With this method the thumb Is wrapped around the bar and then the fingers encircle the thumb. Some one hand dead lifters use a handkerchief to tighten their grip, but this is not legal in making a record attempt with this style of lifting. The back is kept as Hat as possible throughout the lift. After the bar has been gripped securely, the shoulder on the lifting side should be raised as high as possible. From this position the legs are straightened until they are braced. The non-lifting hand is turned during the progress of the lift so that the thumb and fingers are on the outside of the thigh. This permits the holding of the proper position for the count at the completion of the lift.

Should you find that it is possible for you to lift a greater poundage with the bell parallel to your front for record at-tempts, proceed as follows: Stand with the feet shoulder width apart, and under the bell. Bend the knees, and, keeping the back flat, lower the buttocks to the lifting position as the bar is firmly grasped. The non-lifting hand is placed upon the thigh as in the other position. Straighten the legs until the necessary height of the bell is reached; then hold it for the count.

In this lift the only causes for disqualification would be the failure to lift the bell to the height of the knees or to lock the knees. It is permissible for the bell to touch the legs during the lift.

RIGHT HAND DEAD WEIGHT LIFT

LIFT NO. 6.—Identical with left hand dead weight lift except that opposite hand is employed.

PULL OVER AND PRESS ON BACK WITHOUT BRIDGE

Official Definition

LIFT No. 7.—Lie on the floor, back down, with the bar bell within easy reach immediately back o[head. Draw the bar to a position over the chest with the upper arms resting upon the floor. The heels are kept together, the knees straight and the buttocks upon the floor while the lift is in progress. From the starling position the hell is pressed to arm's length overhead.

Method of Performance

Lying upon the floor with barbell directly back of head grasp the bar with the hands equidistant from the center. It

Is easier to pull the bar over if the hands are held somewhat less than shoulder width apart. As the boll is pulled to a position directly over the body, the head is turned to the side and the elbows arc rested upon the floor. Many lifters shift their grip before pressing, finding it easier to press with the hands considerably wider than shoulder width apart. Either position is permissible. The bar is held with a tight grip to prevent it from rolling back upon the fingers, and then the bell is pressed to arm's length overhead. The bell is held for the count. Practice will determine which style of pressing suits you best. Some prefer to keep the hands less than shoulder width apart, pressing with the elbows held close to the body. Others grasp the bar wide and press with the elbows extended out from the body. It will be possible to lock the arms in the shortest possible time if the bell is held back over the face while the lift is in progress.

Causes for Disqualification Are: The bending of the legs, raising of the buttocks or shoulders, and the separation of the heels.

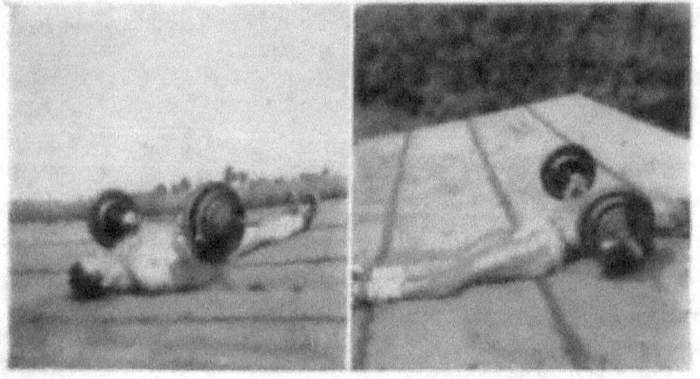

Pull over and press on back without bridge. Posed by Eddie Harrison and John Grimek.

PULL OVER AND PRESS ON BACK WITH BRIDGE

Official Definition

LIFT NO. 8.—Lying on the floor with the center of the bar immediately behind the head the bell shall be brought over the lifter's face until the upper arms rest on the ground. Once the bell clears the line of the sternum where the collar bones meet, the disks shall not again be brought into contact with the floor. Immediately the bell is in the same position as for the "press." then the heels may be brought close to the buttocks, and the forearms inclined forward until the bar rests across the abdomen. From this position the bell may be impelled to arm's length overhead by a quick "bridge" formation, but at no period of the lift shall the shoulders leave the ground. At the conclusion of the lift the arms and legs shall be straight, the buttocks on the floor, and the heels be brought together.

Method of Performance

The bell is pulled over the face in the same manner as in the press on back without bridge. From this position, draw up the feet until the heels are up close against the buttocks. The body is raised upwards and the elbows inclined so that the bar rests across the abdomen. The heels are kept slightly apart, from six inches to a foot being the accepted practice with most lifters.

This style of lifting the bar has often been called the "belly toss." Some men are so flexible that they do all of the lifting with the abdomen, the arms catching and holding the weight only near the completion of the lift. Retaining the bar upon the abdomen, the body is lowered until the buttocks almost touch the floor, then, with a quick raise of the abdomen or toss the bar is thrown from its position across the body backwards over the face. There the lift is finished by a strong pressure from the arms. When the bell is at arm's length, lower the buttocks, straighten the legs, place the heels together and hold the bell for the count.

Cause for Disqualification Is: Not observing the ruling that the bell must not be lowered again when once it has passed the line of the sternum.

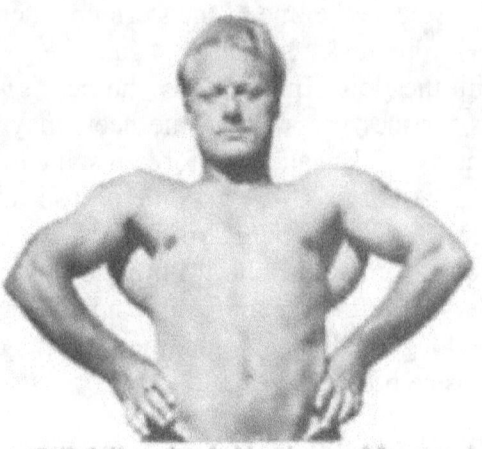

Bill Lilly who holds the world's record on the pull over and press with bridge. He uses the style commonly called "the belly toss."

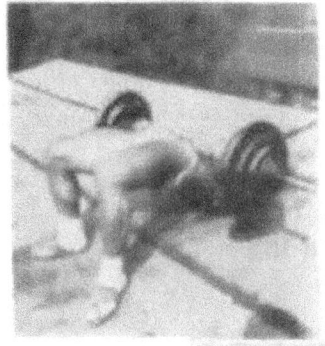
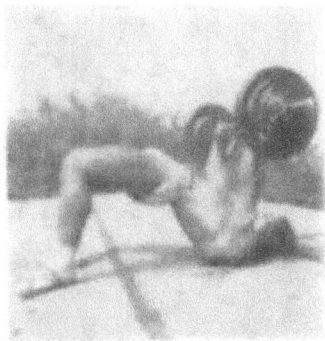
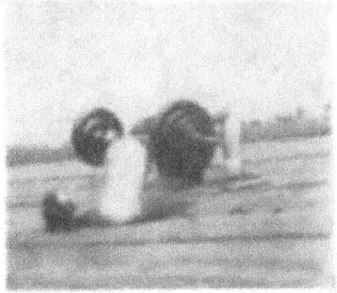

Pull over and press on back with bridge. Grimek and Harrison demonstrating the lift.

PRESS ON BOX OR BENCH

Official Definition

LIFT NO. 9.—Lie upon your back on a bench with feet resting upon the floor. Two boxes which serve the same purpose may be employed. A helper lifts the weight over until it rests upon the lifter's chest. From this position it is pressed to arm's length overhead. No raising of the buttocks or bridging of any sort is permitted.

Method of Performance

If boxes similar to those in which York bar bells are shipped are employed, the lifter can reach back to the bar, ascertaining the correct position by placing his hands at the

129

edge of knurling. From there the assistant lifts the bar over the lifter's chest. Most men can press best in this position with the hands a bit less than shoulder width apart and the elbows held dose to the body while the lift is consummated. The bar is held overhead for the count.

Causes for Disqualification Are: The raising of the buttocks or bridging in any form, during the lift.

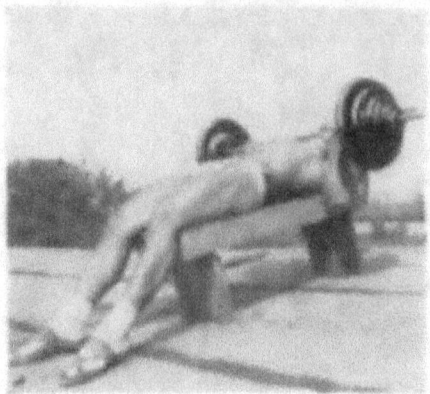

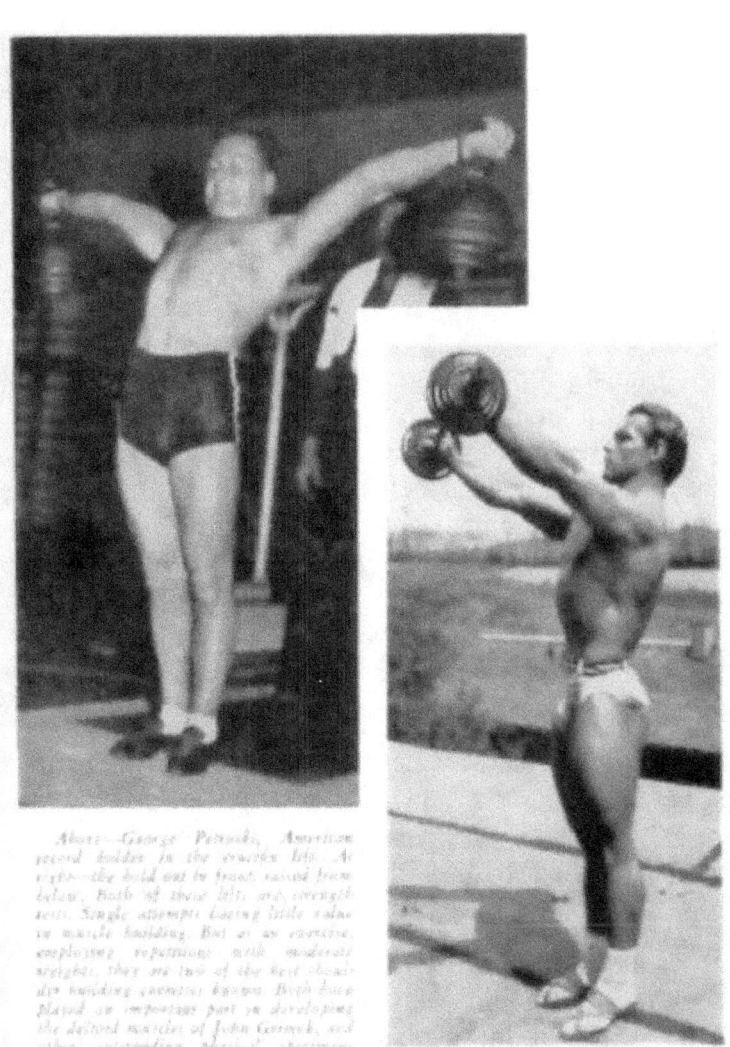

Above—George Petrusak, American record holder in the snatch lift. At right—the hold out in front, raised from below. Both of these lifts are strength tests. Single attempts having little value in muscle building. But as an exercise, employing repetitions with moderate weights, they are two of the best shoulder building exercises known. Both have played an important part in developing the desired muscles of John Germek, and other outstanding physical specimens pictured in this book.

HOLD OUT IN FRONT. RAISED FROM BELOW

Official Definition

Lift No. 10—The bar bell grasped with both hands (knuckles to the front) shall rest at arm's length across the lifter's front, from which position it shall be raised forward steadily until the units are level with the shoulders. Throughout the lift the trunk must not be inclined backwards, forwards or sideways, the shoulders must be kept quite level, the arms and legs straight and the heels together. Seen from the side, the head, back, buttocks and heels should be in one straight line, and the slightest deviation from this line shall be cause for disqualification.

Method of Performance

Most lifters grasp the bar with hands at shoulder width, although if a greater width seems more suitable in the individual case, it is permissible. Lifting the bar with the knuckles front, it rests across the thighs with the arms hanging straight. Tighten or stiffen the body so that it is erect, in line from heel to head. This position must be maintained throughout the lift. With the elbows firmly locked, raise the bell steadily until the arms reach a position at right angles to the body. The count is taken at this position.

The greatest difficulty in performing this lift is to maintain the perpendicular position of the body. The trunk has a tendency to bend backward to balance the weight. To prevent this the shoulders should be carried forward as the lift is started.

Causes for Disqualification Are: The separation of the heels, the failure to keep the body absolutely upright throughout the lift, and not bring the bell to the level of the shoulders for the count.

CRUCIFIX

Official Definition

LIFT No. 11—The dumbells (kettle bells or ring weights) having been taken to arm's length overhead shall be lowered sideways (palms uppermost) until the arms are level, with the shoulders. If ring weights are used, they will not be allowed to rest upon the forearms, but must hang suspended from the rings. Whilst the bells are being lowered, the trunk may be inclined backwards to any extent but the heels must remain together and the arms and legs be kept straight throughout.

Method of Performance

The rules permit a choice of several weights: dumbells, ring weights, or kettle bells. But a little practice will determine that ring weights permit the best performance. Most lifters prefer to use this type of equipment. Lift the bells to arm's length overhead. Turn them so that the knuckles are out; the handles should be held diagonally across the palms. Keeping the elbows straight, lower the arms downward steadily until the arms are at right angles to the body. The count is taken at this position. To avoid dropping the weights against the thigh at the completion of the lift, assistants can grasp them, or you can raise ON the toes a bit, bending the back so that the bells will swing down back of the body.

Causes for Disqualification Are: The separation of the legs, separation of the heels, not bringing the weight entirely in line with the shoulders and not keeping the arms straight throughout the lift.

LATERAL RAISE, STANDING

Official Definition

LIFT NO. 12.—The dumbells (or ring weights) shall be at arm's length by the lifter's sides, from which position they shall be raised sideways knuckles uppermost until the arms arc level with the shoulders. Whilst the bells are being raised, the trunk may be inclined backwards to any extent, but the heels must remain together, and the arms and legs kept straight throughout.

Method of Performance

The bells should be taken from the floor to a position against the sides of the thighs, knuckles out, arms straight. In this lift, as in the crucifix, the lifter has the choice of types of weights to be used. The bells are held up tight in the hand against the base of the thumbs, from which position, keeping the arms straight, they are raised steadily sideways until they reach a position at right angles to the body. The count is taken at this position. The hells can be lowered in the same manner as described in the crucifix, if desired.

Causes for Disqualification Are: The same as those described in performing the crucifix lift.

TWO HANDS SLOW CURL

Official Definition

LIFT NO. 13.— The bar bell grasped (with both hands palms to the front) shall hang at arm's length across the lifter's front, from which position it shall be lifted to the shoulders by bending the forearms completely on the upper arms. Through the lift the trunk must not be inclined backwards, forwards or sideways, the shoulders must be kepi quite level, the legs straight, the heels together. The slightest deviation from this position shall be counted cause for disqualification.

Method of Performance

Grasp the bar a bit more than shoulder width apart, with the palms up. Straighten up with the bell, permitting it to lie against the front of the thigh with the arms straight. A perpendicular line must be maintained from head to heels as the arms are bent until the bell has been brought to a level with the shoulders, at which point the count is taken.

While the body must be kept exactly erect throughout the lift, with no jerking or leaning sideways or back, the rule does not insist that the elbows be kept close to the sides throughout the lift. Some lifters pull the elbows well back as the curl is made; others raise the shoulders, as the arms are curled. The bringing of more muscles into play permits a higher record in this lift.

Causes for Disqualification Are: The separation of the heels, the failure to keep the body absolutely upright throughout the lift and not bringing the bell to the shoulders for the count.

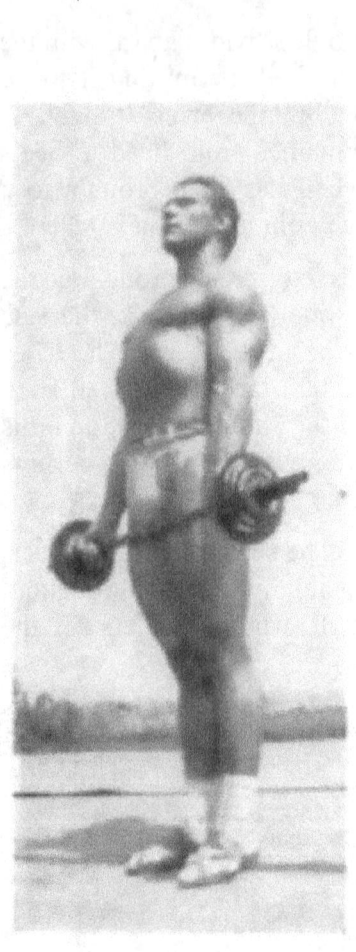
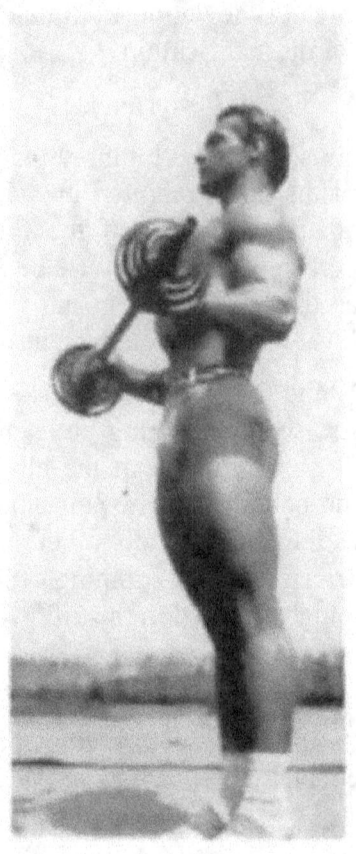

Two hands slow curl. Note at the start, the elbows are locked, the wrists turned back. Like all weight lifting movements best results are obtained by exercising the muscles from the extreme of contraction to the extreme of extension in every movement.

BACK HAND CURL

Official Definition

LIFT NO. 14.—The barbell, grasped with both hands (knuckles to the front), shall hang at arm's length across the lifter's front, from which position it shall be lifted to the shoulders by bending the forearms completely on the upper arms. Throughout the lift the trunk must not be inclined backwards, forwards or sideways: the shoulders must be kept quite level, the legs straight, the heels together. The elbows must be held against the body. The slightest deviation from this position will be counted cause for disqualification.

Method of Performance

Lift the bell from the floor so that it rests across the front of the thighs. Knuckles arc held front and the arms are straight. Tighten or stiffen the body so that it is held firmly erect, in line from head to heel. This position must be maintained throughout the lift. With the elbows held firmly against the body raise the bell forward and up steadily until the bell has been brought to the height of the shoulders. Take the count at this point.

Causes for Disqualification Are: The failure to keep ihe body absolutely upright throughout the lift, any motion which may be considered swinging of the bar, and the removal of the elbows from the sides of the body.

RIGHT HAND CURL

Official Definition

LIFT No. 15. The dumbell (or kettle bell) is grasped with the right hand, palm front. It is brought to a point where it hangs at arm's length across the lifter's front, from which position it shall be lifted to the shoulders by bending the forearm completely on the upper arms. Throughout the lift the trunk must not be inclined backwards, forwards or sideways; the shoulders must be kept quite level, the legs straight, and the heels together.

Method of Performance

It is not difficult to perform either the right or left hand curl by following the instructions of the definition describing the method to be used already offered.

LEFT HAND CURL

LIFT NO. 16.—Similar in all respects to the right hand curl.

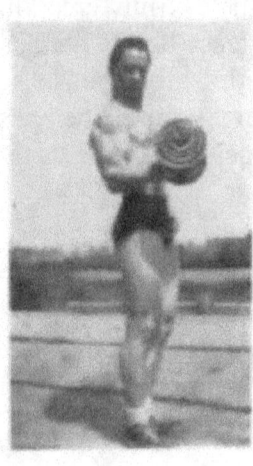
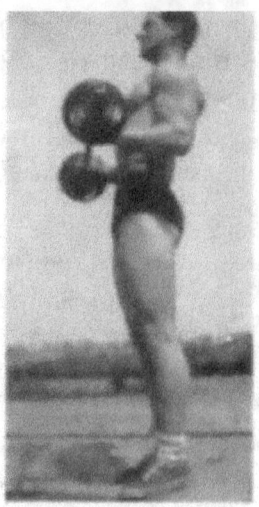

Eddie Harrison of York, performing one hand curl and the back hand curl.

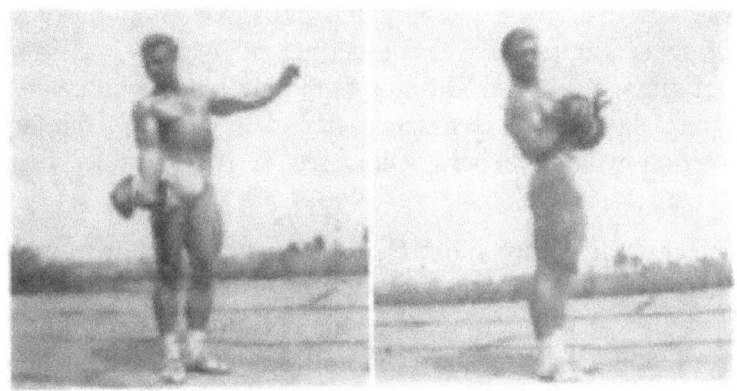

Grimek at the start and finish of a one hand curl.

LEFT HAND MILITARY PRESS

Official Definition

LIFT NO. 17.—The dumbell shall be taken to the shoulder and, after a pause of two seconds, pressed to arm's length overhead. At the commencement of the press the bar shall not be held higher than the top of the sternum where the collar bones meet. During the press from the shoulder the trunk must not be inclined backwards, forwards. or sideways; the shoulders must be kept quite level, the legs straight, the heels together, the head held erect with the eyes looking directly to the front, the slightest deviation from the erect position bring counted cause for disqualification, hi taking the bell to the shoulder either one or two hands may be used. In the performance of this lift the use of a bar bell or ring weight is not permitted.

Method of Performance

The dumbell should be placed upon the floor at right angles to the body, then standing astride the bell, grasp the handle with the hand close to the inside front disk. The bell should then be swung to arm's length. Now assume the military position with the heels together, the body perpendicular from head to heel, at the same time extending the non-lifting arm to the side al shoulder height. While some lifters preliminary to one arm military pressing will swing the bell to the shoulder, it is much easier to assume the military position when the hell is lowered to the shoulder from above.

The chief difficulty in one hand military pressing is to resist the tendency to bend to the side or back. From the position as shown in illustration, press the bell upwards steadily to arm's length overhead. Take the count at this position. Forcing the bell to lean backwards will assist tin- locking of the arm while still maintaining the military position.

Causes for Disqualification Are: The bending of the legs, the separating of die heels, starting the press with the bell held above the sternum, failing to pause for two seconds at the shoulder level or after the bell is overhead, or failing to keep the body exactly upright throughout the lift.

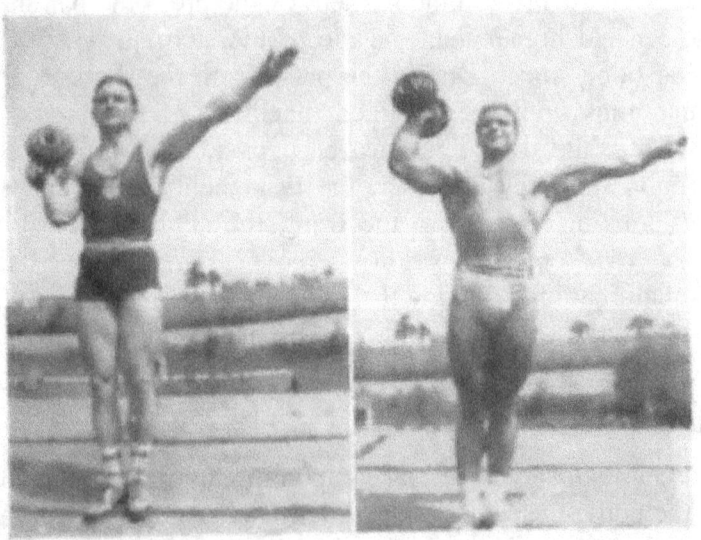

Right hand military press as performed by world's champion Johnny Terpak and Grimek.

RIGHT HAND MILITARY PRESS

LIFT NO. 18.—Performed exactly the same as the left hand military press except that the right hand is employed.

LEFT HAND SIDE PRESS

Official Definition

LIFT NO. 19.—The bar is brought to a position somewhat similar to that of the bent press except that the lifting arm must be held free from the body. The heels must be held on a line and not more than shoulder width apart. Holding the arm and bell away from the body the weight is pressed to arm's length overhead. The trunk may be bent as much as possible but the legs must remain absolutely straight throughout the entire lift. The non-lifting arm must be held free from the body and can not be employed to assist in any manner.

Method of Performance

The bell is lifted to the shoulder with both hands, if preferred, the feet are placed in line, the knees locked firmly and then the bell is lifted free from the body. In cleaning the bell to the shoulder the bell should be grasped with the lifting hand at the right side of the bar's knurling, or if an unknurled bar is used, at least one inch to the right of center. Then a back hang should be induced as the bar is turned around in line with the feet. The feet should point in the direction in which the trunk will fall. The legs must remain straight. 'The shoulder is lifted high; the trunk is bent far to the side as the arm strongly presses the weight overhead until the arm is locked. As in the bent press the hip should be forced well to the side, and although it does not support the weight as in the bent press, the bending of the trunk is made easier. When the arm is locked, rise to the erect position, trunk perpendicular, with the non-lifting arm held at shoulder height to the side. Take the count in this position.

Causes for Disqualification Are: Any failure to follow the rules just enumerated, not holding the bell free from the body, bending the legs during the lift, heels too far apart, or any support supplied by the non-lifting arm.

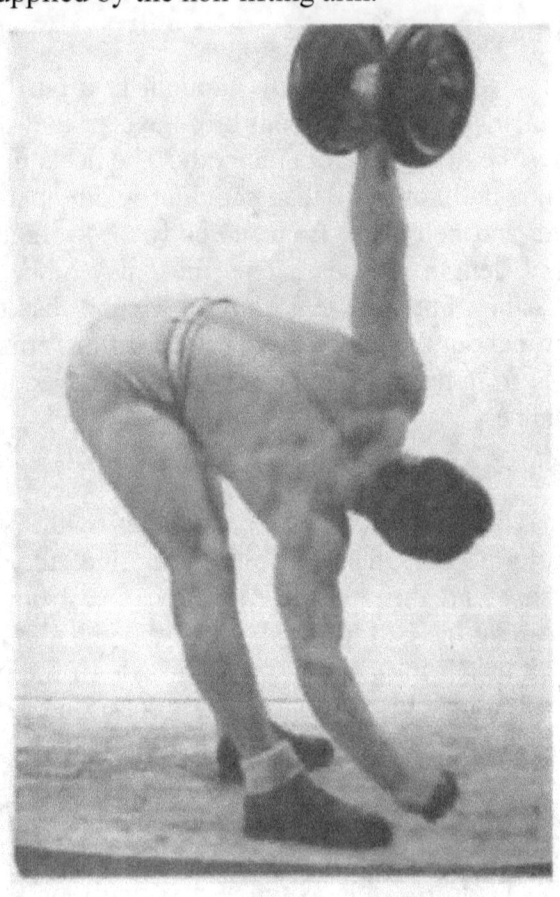

Eddie Harrison at the low point in the one hand side press. Eddie is a great all around athlete, acrobat, tumbler and balancer as well as a champion lifter.

Lift No. 20.—Same procedure as for left hand side press.

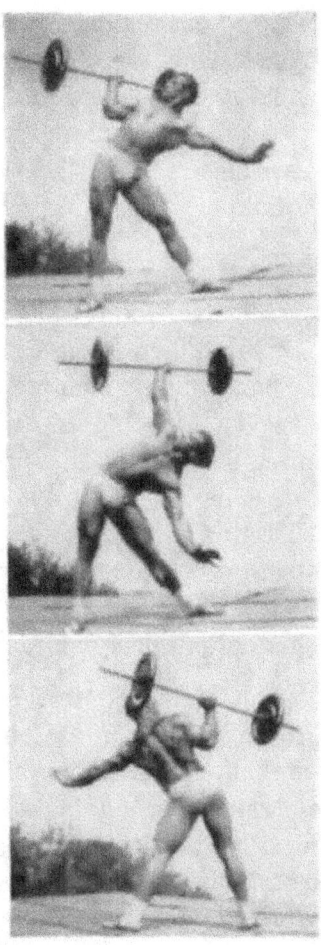

John Grimek, one of the world's best side and bent pressers, demonstrating his form in the side press. His record in the bent press is 268 pounds.

DEEP KNEE BEND WITH FEET FLAT

Official Definition

Lift No. 21.—Place bar upon shoulders. It is permissible to have it lifted there by assistants. The feet can be held either close together or wide apart as the lifter prefers. Lower until the full squat is reached, then come back to the erect position without assistance from the hands: At the completion of the lift hold the weight for the count of two.

Method of Performance

The weight may be rocked to the shoulders by the lifter, taken from a trestle or lifted there by assistants. The bar is held in place with the hands. Some men prefer to wrap their arms around the bar. The placing of the feet is most important. Place them in the position that practice proves to be best for you. While some men deep knee bend with not more than a foot separating the feet, there arc others who prefer to stand with them very wide apart. In this latter style it is easier to keep the back flat. A flat back is most important in reaching record or near record performances.

Lower until the full squat is reached, then raise to the erect position. There are some lifters who use one hand on their thigh to assist in rising, but this is not permissible. It is best to take several deep breaths before going into the low squat position. Some men exhale rapidly as the body is lowered, catch a quick breath at the lowest point and regain the erect position where they breathe deeply again. But for a single attempt the several preliminary breaths should be sufficient.

Causes for Disqualification Are: A rounded back during the lift is not cause for disqualification, but it adds to the difficulty of performing a heavy deep knee bend. Not going into the lowest possible squat, or assisting with the hands in rising are causes for disqualification. The feet must be on a line, with the knees straight and the back erect when the count Is taken.

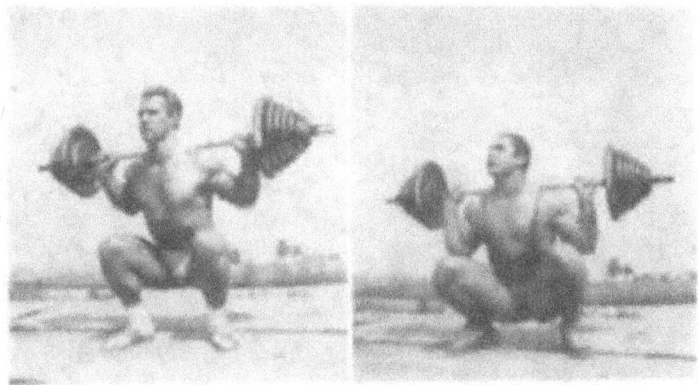

Deep knee bend with flat feet. Note the straight back and very low position of both Grimek and Stanko in these illustrations.

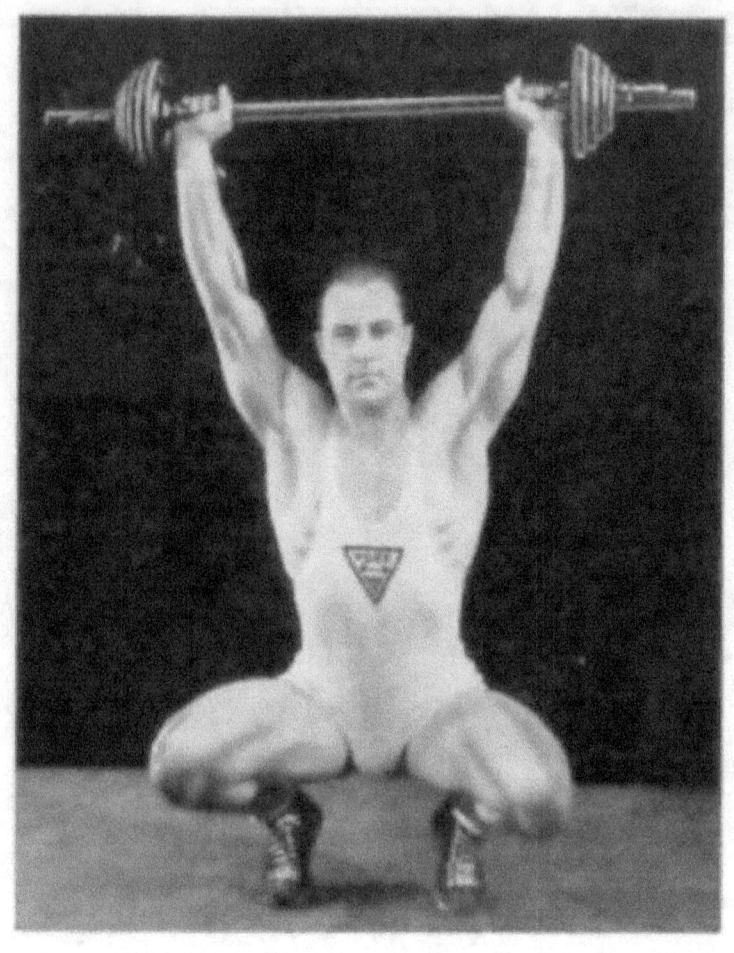

Gord Venables, all around athlete, associate editor Strength and Health magazine, weight lifting champion of North America, demonstrating how the deep knee bend with weight overhead is performed.

DEEP KNEE BEND ON TOES. HOLDING WEIGHT OVERHEAD

Official Definition

LIFT No. 22.—The weight can be taken to arm's length overhead in any way the lifter prefers. From a starting position with heels in line, the knees are bent and the body lowered as far as possible, meanwhile holding the bar bell at arm's length overhead. The lift is complete and the count taken after the lifter is erect, still holding the weight overhead, standing with the feet on a line.

Method of Performance

Stand in the position you have found to be most suitable in your own ease for cleaning, snatching, or pulling the weight to the shoulders. Practice will show you the width of grip which works best for you in this lift. The majority will prefer a very wide grip as this enables the lifter to better maintain his balance as he goes into the low squat position. Lift the weight to arm's length overhead, stand with the heels on a line, the toes a comfortable distance apart, which is usually an angle of about forty-five degrees. As you lower the body, the back must lie kept fiat to maintain balance. The heels will rise from the floor. Turn the knees well out as this will not only assist you in maintaining balance but will add to the development you obtain from the practice of this lift.

This particular movement requires considerable balance and is made a part of the lifts contained in this book, as it builds balance, strength in muscles which are not brought fully into play in other movements, and assists the lifting specialist in becoming proficient at the two hands snatch squat style if that is the method which permits him to lift the greatest poundage. When you rise from the full squat, hold the weight overhead and the feet on a line for the count. Breathing is the same in this exercise as already described in the deep knee bend with flat feet.

ROWING MOTION

Official Definition

Lift No. 23.—With the legs straight and the upper body at right angles to them, the bar must be lifted from the dead hang position at arm's length until it touches the chest. No jerking or movement of the upper body is permitted. Hold the bar against the chest for the count at the completion of the lift.

Method of Performance

Stand with the legs a comfortable distance apart, usually shoulder width. Practice will show you the width of grip that Is best in your particular case. You will have noticed that I frequently make this statement. No two men arc exactly alike in construction and body leverage. Some can exert force better with a close grip than wide, either in two hands pressing, two hands snatching or cleaning, even in the deep knee bend with close or wide spacing of the feet, and some men can perform their best rowing motion with the hands spaced about shoulder width apart, while others prefer a much wider grip. Regardless of the spacing of the hands the performance of the lift is the same. The legs must be held straight, the upper body inclined forward at right angles to the legs. After gripping the bar with the hand grip that you prefer, let it hang for at least two seconds with arms straight. You are then ready to lift the weight. It must be pulled to the chest without motion of the upper body— entirely by the muscles of the arms and the upper back. In practice, some men place their head upon the back of a chair which prevents movement of the head and upper back.

Causes for Disqualification Are: Not starting with the bell hanging downward at arm's length, any movement of the upper body or raising of the head when the bar is pulled to chest, failing to hold it for two seconds for the count in that position at the completion of the lift.

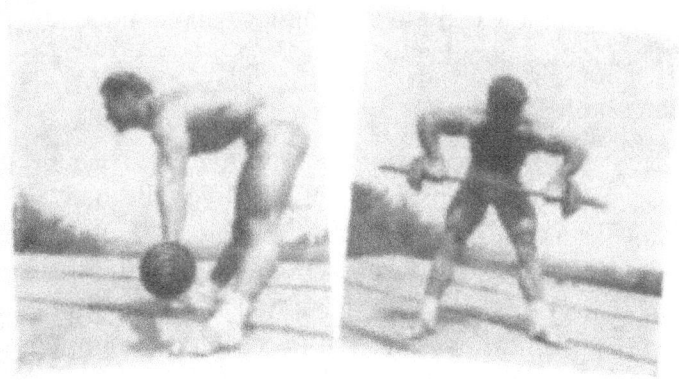

The rowing motion. Correct illustrating the start and the half way point. Position at the completion of the rowing motion, arms, wrists, elbows and. Many men perform this movement with the arms about shoulder width apart keeping the elbows near the body.

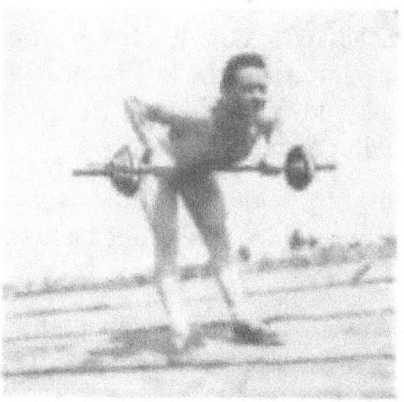

LEG PRESS

Official Definition

Lift No. 24.—Lie upon the back on a floor. No special equipment to raise the lower back is permitted. Either place or have lifted to the bottoms of your feet the bar bell you intend to lift. Then lower the legs and the bar bell to the lowest possible position. The judges must determine just how low is the lowest position with the average individual.

149

Then press the weight to straight legs above the body. Hold it there lor the count.

Method of Performance

After lying flat upon your back on the ground pull up the legs so that they are held directly over the body. While many lifters are able to place 300 or more pounds upon their feet unassisted, when a high poundage is reached it should be lifted upon the feet by assistants. In practicing this movement, if it is desired to place the weight upon the feel unassisted, the liar should lw pulled over and pressed with bridge as described in making that lift. First one foot and then the other is placed under the bar. When your

training mates place the bar upon the feet, hold the legs straight overhead. When the weight is properly balanced, it is lowered until it reaches the lowest possible position. Men with large legs and big bodies must space the feet wider apart than smaller men.

The weight must be held in the low position for at least two seconds, then pressed to straight legs and again held for the count of two.

Causes for Disqualification Are: Failing to lower the weight to the lowest possible position, failure to hold it there for the count of two, failure to have the legs locked when the bell Is overhead, and to hold the weight there for two seconds.

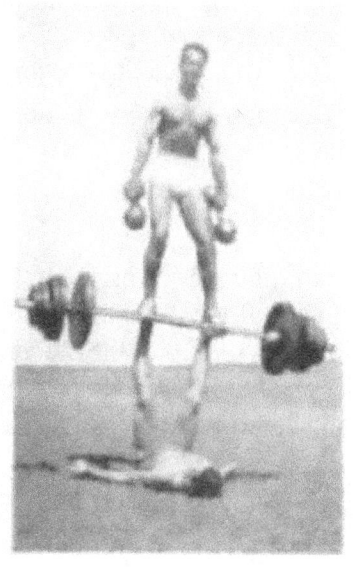

LEG BICEPS CURL

Definition of the Lift

LIFT No. 25. The lifter lies upon the floor fat e down. The lifting apparatus consists of a pair of iron boots, in the groove of which a bar bell has been placed. The feet should be spaced shoulder width apart. The legs are extended so that the toes rest upon the floor. When the signal to lift is given, the legs are curled until the weight is directly over the body. There it is held for the count of two. In the process of making the lift the body must remain flat upon the floor.

Method of Performance

This is a great developing exercise and is practiced nearly everywhere that weight lifting is known. While it can best be performed with a pair of York Iron Boots, owing to the ease with which the barbell can lie plated in the groove (a patented feature found only with tin- York Iron Boots), any similar appliance can BE used. The barbell thrust through the grooves of the iron boots is loaded to the desired poundage. Then the lifter lies in the supine position, which of course means with face down, upon a bench or table. The legs are extended. When the signal to lift is given the weights are curled steadily until they are directly over the body; there they are held for the count.

Causes for Disqualification Are: Failure to straighten the legs at the start of the lift, the raising of the buttocks or any part of the body except the lower legs from the bench, boxes or table during the progress of the lift, failing to hold the weight over the body with legs at right angles at completion of lift.

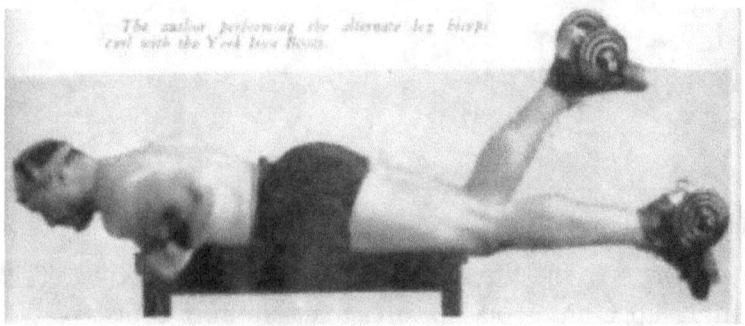

HALF KNEE BEND

Description of the Lift

LIFT No. 26.—The bar is placed upon the lifter's shoulders. either taken from a trestle or lilted there by assistants. The body braced, the knees straight, feet the preferable distance apart. When the signal the clapping of the referee's hands is given, the lifter will lower his body not less than one foot. Upon the return to the erect position the count is taken.

Method of Performance

This lift is included among the record program of lifts because the body must be taught to handle really heavy poundages if the maximum of strength and development is to be obtained. As specified by the rules, the weight can be placed upon the shoulders either by assistants or from a trestle. The weight should be carried low on the back of the shoulders, the chin lifted slightly, the back flattened to the extent of being slightly concave. The body must be lowered at least one foot and then brought back to the starting position, at which point the count is taken.

This lift has especial merit in imparting power, spring and energy to the muscles of the knees. It will add pounds to the quirk lifter's total.

Cause for Disqualification Is: Not lowering the body sufficiently.

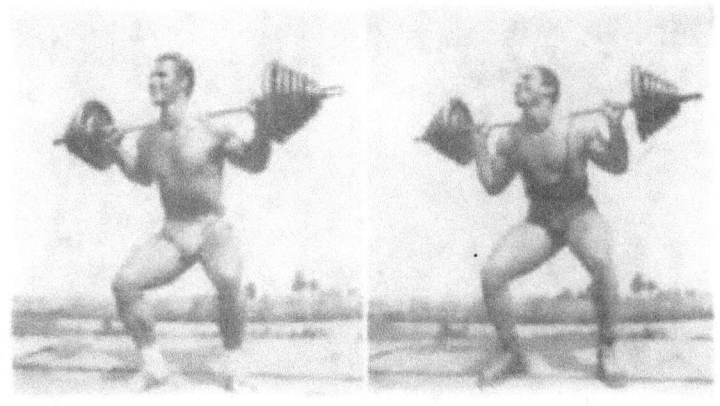

The half knee bend. The movement imparts great power and spring to the legs. Advanced bar bell men now employ at least 600 pounds in this lift.

STRADDLE LIFT

Definition of the Lift

LIFT No. 27. In this lift the bar bell can be placed upon a pair of boxes not more than one foot in height. The lifter straddles the bar and baring one hand in front and the other to the rear, lifts the weight until the legs and back are straight, at which point the count is taken.

Place the bar upon the low boxes. Stand above the bar with the feet about eighteen inches apart and toes turned outward. By bending the knees, lower the body until the bar may be grasped with one hand in front of body, -one in back, palms of hands toward body. Keeping the back flat and exerting most of the power with the legs, straighten the legs and the body. When the erect position as described is reached the count of two should be taken. A great amount of weight can be employed in this style of lifting. Great strength in muscles, ligaments and tendons will be developed.

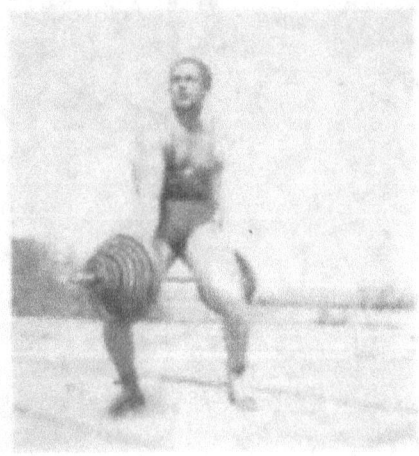

The Straddle Lift, an other movement in which great poundages can be lifted.

THE LEG RAISE

Official Definition

LIFT NO. 28. Lying flat upon the back, the weights are fastened to the lifter's feet preferably with the iron boots

154

and bar bell. Keeping the upper body and bullocks upon the floor, the legs, remaining straight throughout, are raised until they are directly above the body. At this point the count is taken.

Method of Performance

As is evident from die description and practice of this lift, it is one that will develop a powerful external and internal waistline. Its developing action is slightly different from the abdominal raise, already described, and for that reason is particularly beneficial when practiced in conjunction with the abdominal raise. The same assembly used in the leg biceps curl should BE employed. The York iron boots serve best. But any similar assembly, even tying weights to the feet, may be employed in the practice of, or performance of, this lift.

It will be necessary to hold some weighty object with the hands back of head to keep the upper body from rising when the attempt is made to raise the legs. The body must remain in contact with the floor, the legs remain straight throughout the lift .is the weight is slowly and steadily raised from its position upon the floor to a point directly over the BODY. When this position is reached the count is taken.

Raising any part of the body except the legs from the floor, the failure to keep the legs straight throughout the lift and for the count of two when the legs are overhead.

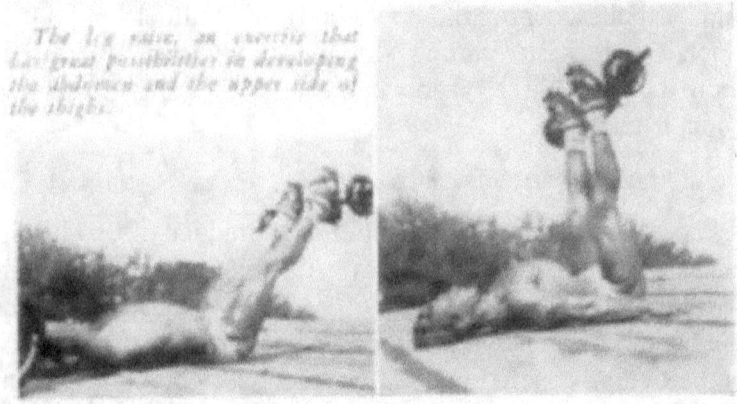

The leg raise, an exercise that has great possibilities in developing the abdomen and the upper side of the thighs.

BEND OVER

Official Definition

Lift No. 29. The weight placed across the shoulders, and with the legs held perfectly straight, the body is inclined forward until it reaches a position at right angles

Method of Performance

It is optional with the lifter as to how the weight should be placed across the shoulders. He can clean and jerk it to its position behind neck, he can take it from a pair of trestles or have it lifted into place by assistants. The feel are placed about shoulder width apart, the knees locked, the back held as flat as possible, the head held back as the low forward position Is reached. The back kept flat, the legs straight, the weight is lifted to the upright position at which point the count is taken. This lift is commonly called the "good morning" exercise, as its practice is similar to a person bowing a good morning greeting.

Causes for Disqualification Are: The failure to keep the legs straight, failure to reach the position with the upper body parallel to the floor as the legs remain at right angles to it, failure to hold the weight for the count when the upright position is regained.

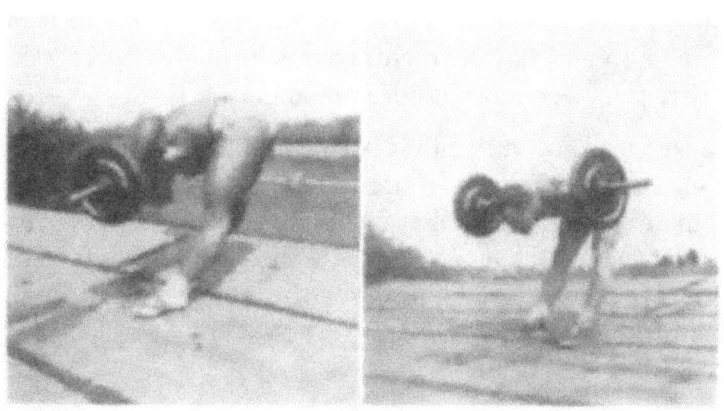

The bend over or Good Morning exercise. Requires great strength and flexibility in the lower back. Builds strength and unusual suppleness to bring into action the huge muscles of the lower back.

ALTERNATE PRESS, TEN REPETITIONS

Official Definition

Lift No. 30.—Two dumbells are swung to a position at shoulder height. From this position the arms are alternately pressed to arm's length overhead and in turn lowered. A weight which can be properly handled ten repetitions, five with each hand, is required. The weight must be lowered to at least the level of the shoulder and extended to straight arm's length overhead. The count is taken with both dumbells held overhead.

Method of Performance

Place the dumbells upon the door at right angles to the body. Grasp one in each hand, with the hand (lose to the forward inside plate. Swing them in one quick movement to shoulder height. From this position press the left arm to straight arm's length overhead. As the right arm is pressed

157

to the same position the left is lowered to shoulder height. This movement is continued until the necessary ten repetitions are made, the weight held overhead for the count of two. A rocking motion is permissible as the bells are pressed. The legs must remain locked throughout but movement of the shoulders and upper body is permissible. This is a good development exercise—builds the pressing ability from a somewhat different angle.

Causes for Disqualification Are: Failure to start the weight from shoulder height, failure to straighten the arm entirely in the overhead position at the completion of each one arm press, bending the legs throughout the lift, or failing to hold the two dumbells overhead for the count of two at the completion of the lift.

Advanced Lifts

Lift No. 31.—The bar bell shall be taken clean to the shoulders in one continuous movement, and come to rest upon the upper chest. The recovery from the " pull in," preparatory for the press, must be speedy and continuous. At the commencement of the press the bar shall not be held higher than the sternum or collar bone, and the leet if separated must be on the same plane, placed no wider apart than sixteen inches, with knees firmly braced, and body and head held in an upright position. During the press from the chest, no lowering of the bell, shrugging, or jerking, sagging or turning of the trunk, movement of the feet or bending of the legs shall be permitted, and the movement must be a steady press to arm's length with the shoulders kept level throughout.

The referee shall insist upon a pause of two seconds at the shoulders, and again at the conclusion of the lift. In both cases he shall indicate the conclusion of the short compulsory pause by a sharp dap with the hands. Lifters who are unable to rest the bar on their chests must inform the referee of that fact before beginning the lift. For this class of lifter the starting position of the press shall be a point in front of the lifter at the point of the sternum where it meets the collar bone.

Method of Performance The bell is drawn from the floor to the point on the chest where experience has proven that the individual lifter can press best. Most lifters ran pull the weight to the shoulders without moving the feet. There are two distinct styles of pressing which suit individuals of various types. The first and most commonly used is to make the start of the pre s with the bar about the level of

159

the breast bone. The bar 's grasped usually slightly wider than the inside edge of the knurling on the standard bars, so that the elbows are turned in toward the body. The bar lays well back on the fingers.

When the signal to press is given, there must be no lowering of the bell. Press as fast as possible. While formerly there was a rule that the press must be made slowly -in fact at one time the lifter was required to keep pace with the rising of the referee's finger- -it is now permitted to press as fast as desirable, just so the rules arc followed—no movement of the knees, shrugging or sagging in the beginning, bending or twisting of the body, no movement of the feet.

The two hands press variously termed Olympic Press and Military Press was most commonly called the latter, for it is necessary that the body he held erect throughout and that the lifter look straight to the front.

The other method of pressing is started with the bar resting on the sternum and the deltoids. The elbows arc held high and away from the body during the press. With this method it is possible to give the bar a very fast start without giving cause for disqualification. The distance to press is also much shorter. It is easier to complete a heavy press with the wide grip employed by most lifters who use this style.

Causes for Disqualification Are: The failure to hold the feet on line during the press, any movement of the feet, raising of the heel or toe, losing of the balance and a possible short step forward to maintain equilibrium, bending of the knees, starting to press with the bell held higher than the sternum this for those lifters who can not hold the bar on the chest (seldom, however, is a lifter found who can not lay the bar 011 chest if he learns to press with a wider than shoulder width grip)—failure to wait two seconds for the referee's signal to press, stopping of the upward progress of the lift at any stage of the press —although the motion can he fast, it must be continuous any change from the starting position of the press. While it is permissible to start with a slight curve in the back, this position must be maintained throughout. Back bending is one of the most common causes for disqualification; the failure to hold the bell until the referee gives his signal that the lift is completed.

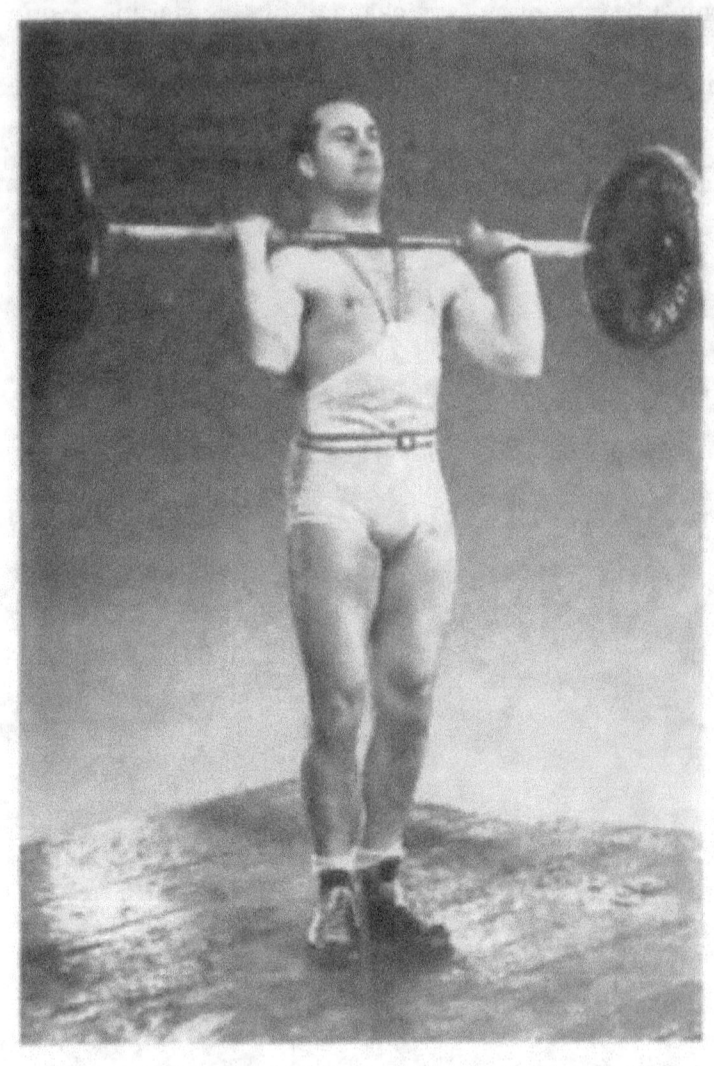

The method of pressing used by Gord Venables. The elbows are held well forward, the weight on top of the shoulders. His record in this lift is 245 pounds.

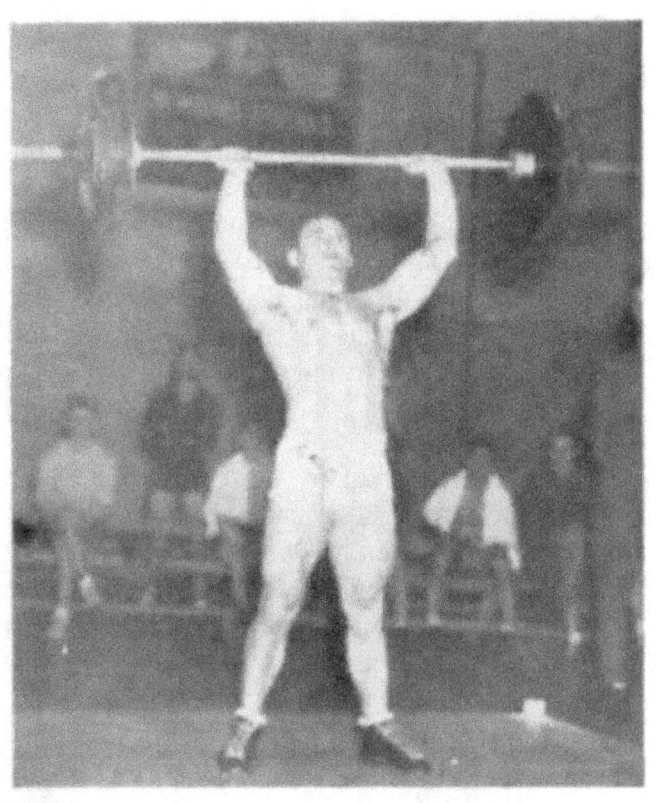

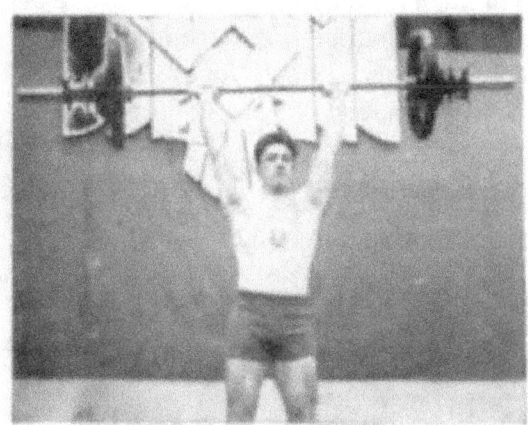

Above: Tony Petrolino, of Chicago, about to complete a heavy military press. He is one of the nation's best pressers. Richter, of Vienna, official holder of world's records, completing a military press.

TWO HANDS PRESS BEHIND NECK

LIFT No. 32.—The bar bell is lifted clean In the chest, then lifted and lowered to a position behind the neck where it rests across the shoulders. The feet must be held in line, either heels together or not more than sixteen inches apart. The bell is then pressed overhead from this position to arm's length. The trunk must be held erect during the press from the shoulders, and there must be no moving of the neck. The trunk shall be erect, the arms and legs straight, the heels together at the conclusion of the lift.

Method of Performance

Clean the weight to the chest in the usual manner. It is permissible to jerk the weight up and over the head with a sudden dipping and straightening of the knees. It is lowered to a position across the shoulders. If the feet have been moved in jerking the bell overhead, be sure that they are in line at this stage of the lift, as you are about to start pressing. The press may he made as rapidly as desired, but there must be 110 jerking or movement of the legs at the start of the press. The movement must be continuous as the bell is pressed to arm's length. The bar is kept as close to the back of the head as possible during the first stage of the lift, then it is allowed to come forward, directly over the head or in front of head if the lifter prefers.

Causes for Disqualification Are: Movement of the feet during the progress of the lift, jerking with the legs at the start of the lift, back In-nding during the lift.

TWO HANDS REPETITION PRESS

Lift No. 33.—At least five repetitions must be performed, coinciding with the rules of correct military pressing.

Method of Performance

This lift is designed to improve pressing ability. It is essential that the details of performance as outlined in the two hands military press BE followed throughout. Through practice the lifter will determine the poundage with which he is most likely to correctly perform five repetitions when making record attempts. There is just as much cause for disqualification on the last press or two if the proper position is not maintained even if the first few presses were made in perfect style. Records will be allowed in this lift just ;is in the lifts consisting of only a single attempt.

Causes for Disqualification Are: Any deviation of the rules as outlined in performing the two hands military press.

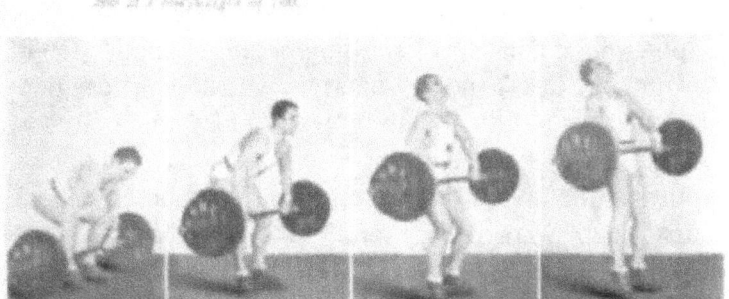

The two hands snatch as performed by Johnny Terpak. Johnny holding middleweight and light heavyweight American record, having snatched 268 at a bodyweight of 180.

TWO HANDS SNATCH

LIFT No. 34.—'The bar bell shall be taken from the ground to outstretched arm's length overhead in one continuous movement. In fixing the bell the legs may be bent to any extent, but to lock the arms by an obvious push shall be counted cause for disqualification. The distance between the hands shall be a matter for the lifter's discretion, but they may not move or slide along the bar once a grip has been taken.

In the recovery from the lunge, dip or squat, care must be taken to resume the erect position speedily in continuous movement. Any delay in the recovery will be counted cause for disqualification, at the conclusion of the lift the neck shall be erect with legs firmly braced, and feet, if separated, placed not wider than sixteen inches apart and held for two seconds until the referee has given a sharp clap with both hands.

Method of Performance

There are almost as many variations in performing this great lift as there are weight lifters. Long practice will de-termine for each man the style that is best suited to hi;, physique and temperament. There are two distinct styles-the split, which consists of splitting or sliding the feet apart, one front, one back, and the squat, in which the lifter's body is lowered to a full squatting position as the bell goes overhead. The squat style is used most by Continental Europeans, the split by the French, British and Egyptians. In this country there are and have been a few good squatters but the majority use the split which is the safer style. It is possible for some men to make a greater record with the squat style but too often there are three failures and the lifter loses his chance at the championship being staged. At present the world's featherweight record is held by Terry of U. S. A., a splitter; the world's lightweight record by Shams, the Egyptian who uses the split style; the middleweight record by Touni, the Egyptian, a splitter; the light-heavy record by Fritz Haller of Germany, a splitter; the heavyweight record by Ronald Walker of England, also a splitter. Records have been held at various times by men using the squat style, but they have in turn been supplanted by " splitters "—good proof that this style, which is most reliable, also permits the greatest poundage to be lifted overhead. There are some men, notably those with comparatively long bodies and shorter legs, who ran squat more easily than they can split and who lack most favorable leverage in the pull up for the split style who may do better with squatting. Practice will prove to every ambitious lifter the style that is bat suited for hint.

Following is the style I prefer and believe to be suited for most lifters. The dive and hook ran easily be mastered and permits the greatest poundage to be elevated. Some few men will prefer to start with the heels together, the knees turned well out as the body is bent to go for the weight. But most can lift best with the feet a comfortable distance apart. It's possible to arrive at the proper position in grasping the bar from a start with the legs erect, but the majority will find it best to stand with a slight bend of the knees and the small of the hack held well in. In going for the bell until perfection of style is attained, permitting rapid movement throughout, a slow dive is best. Keeping the bark flat, the head well up, the buttocks low, bend down and grasp the bar. Some lifters prefer a very wide grip, but a number of the record holders grasp the bar only six to ten inches front the inside of the knurling on the International Olympic type bar. While it's necessary in tills position to pull the weight a bit higher to lock the arms, a great deal more pull is possible. Men with very good grips will not find it necessary to use the hook grip, which consists of wrapping the fingers around the thumb, which has already encircled the bar; but the majority will find a hard strong pull more possible with the hook grip. The arms arc straight as the bar is grasped. The feet are so placed that the shins will just touch the bar as the body is bent to grasp the bar.

When the correct starting position has been achieved, the lifter who has been concentrating on a long hard pull, mentally determining to pull the bar to the highest possible point, commencing the lift. The arms are held straight at the

167

beginning of the lift, as connecting links only. The powerful back and legs give the bar its initial impetus. With every ounce of your strength pull the bar upward, keeping it close to the chest as it rises. Pull it as high as you can. During the lift the hands are turned in toward the body somewhat, and as the bell reaches its highest point and the lifter splits the feet—one forward, one back—the elbows are brought front, the hands turned back and the bell will be supported with locked arms. A vicious second pull will greatly assist you in getting a commendable poundage overhead.

While there are variations in splitting,—some few who pull the bell so far back that it is not necessary to move the front feet; some who step much farther forward than the distance they move the rear foot back,—it's well to remember that a straight line is the shortest distance between the bell's starting point on the floor and the overhead position at the finish of the lift. So pull it straight up and step well forward.

In splitting it's important that the majority of the weight be on the front foot. In fact the movement is so balanced that it is not unlike the position of a one-legged squat, with the back leg serving merely as a support. With this balance it's much easier to rock under a heavy snatch if need be.

The lifter must immediately rise from the low position as soon as the bell is overhead. It is best to do this by holding the rear leg stationary and moving the front leg back. Most lifters step forward with the left leg, but it is immaterial which leg goes front in two hand lifting.

Another variation of the split starts from what is familiarly called the "get set style." With this method of lifting usually a very wide grip of the hands is employed. The hook grip is most often used and the bar gripped as far apart as the distance between the plates will permit. With a very wide grip it is not neccessary to pull the bar so high to fix it at arm's length; neither is it possible to obtain much pull from the arms and shoulders—the real work being done first by the legs and later by the back.

Of our American champions who have acquitted themselves so well in international competition, Terry, who officially holds the world's record in the two hands snatch, employs a very wide grip, as does Steve Stanko who made the world's highest snatch in the world's championship at Vienna. But Terlazzo, who has also hoisted world's record poundages, and Terpak, who has made the world's best snatch for a man of his weight 260 at a normal body weight of less than 160 pounds—and Davis, who has snatched 267, employ a rather close grip. It's evident that various lifters arc suited for slight variations in the style, and practice will determine which style is best for them.

Some men who use the get set style start with the legs already bent, but there are others who momentarily straighten the legs, while grasping the bar, to obtain some rebound as they exert their pull back of the bar.

There are also two distinct styles of squatting with the bar: A nearly erect position when the squat is reached for those men who are suited for it, with the hands held just a bit more than shoulder width apart, and much wider; hand grip with the body well forward as the weight is fixed overhead and the arms well back. This latter method is more suited for the average lifter who wishes to learn the squat style. The illustrations which accompany this lift I believe will show you better than words just how the best men perform the two hands snatch.

Causes for Disqualification Are: The shifting of the hands as the bell goes overhead, pressing out the weight when the bar is overhead—the bell must go to straight arm's length in one continuous movement——failure to recover from the low position immediately.

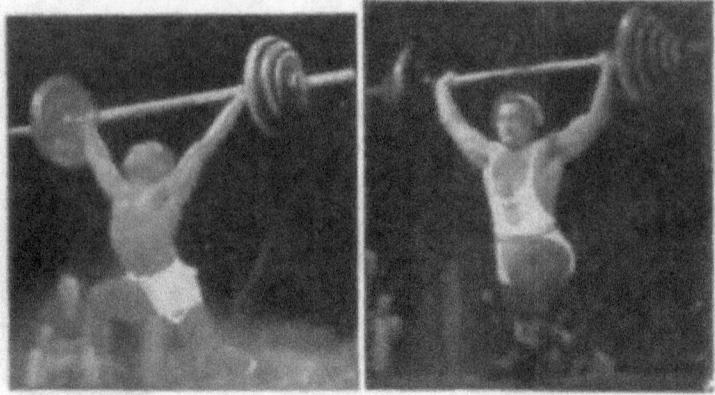

John Terry, who officially holds the record in his bodyweight class at
215 pounds, Steve Stanko, who made the highest two hands snatch in the
world's championships in Vienna.

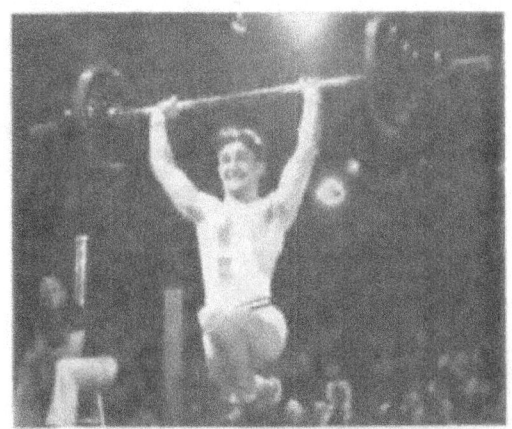

Johnny Terpak matches 231 in the world's championship team match with the German lifter.

Stanley Kratkowski, who held the middleweight two hands snatch record for five years, completing a heavy snatch.

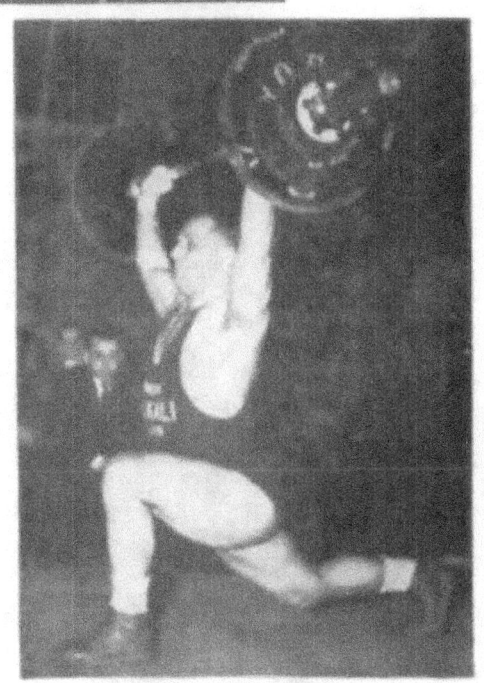

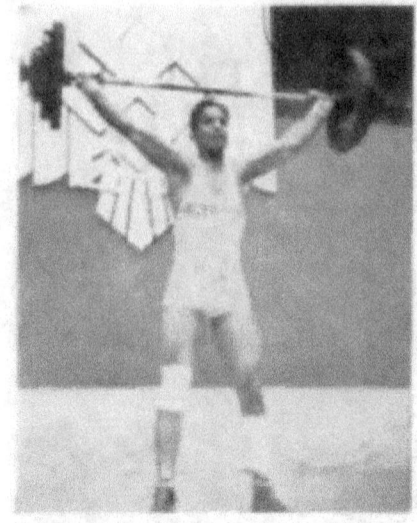

Shams, the Egyptian, who officially holds the world's record 148 pound class, at 248 pounds. Note the very wide grip.

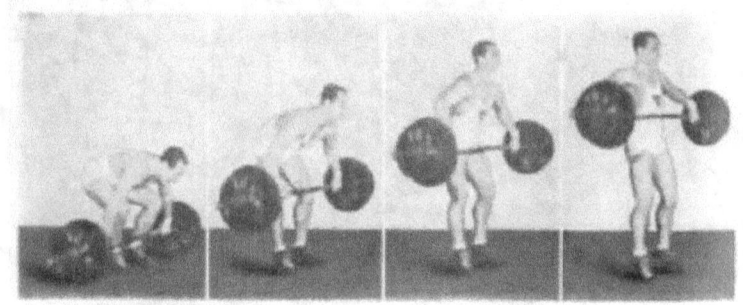

Good Venables' style in the two hands snatch. He uses rather a wide grip and leans well forward.

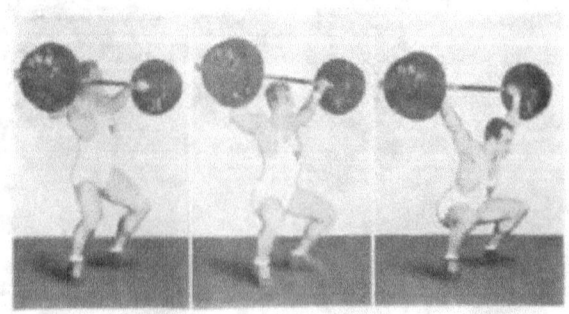

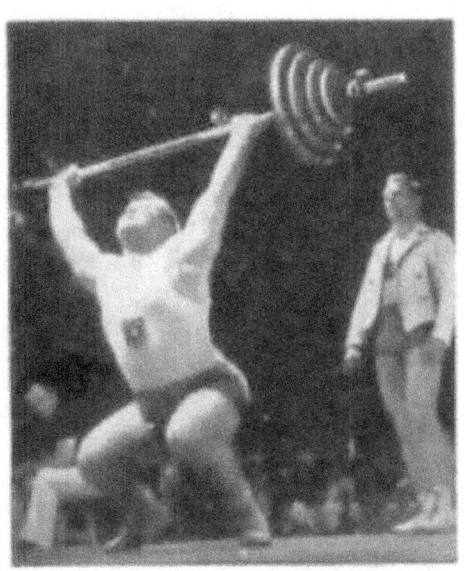

Ma n g e r of Germany, two hands snatching with the squat style on toes. While a good snatcher, he is far below the world's record in this lift. Ismayr, the German captain, is back of Manger ready to catch the weight should he lose balance.

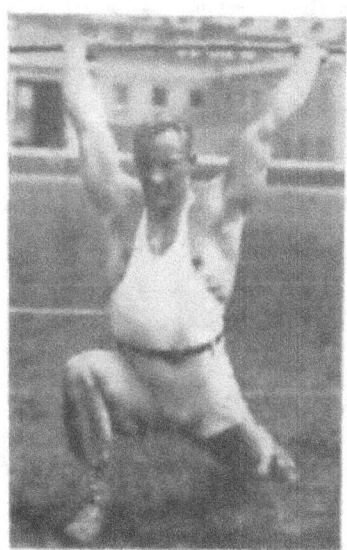

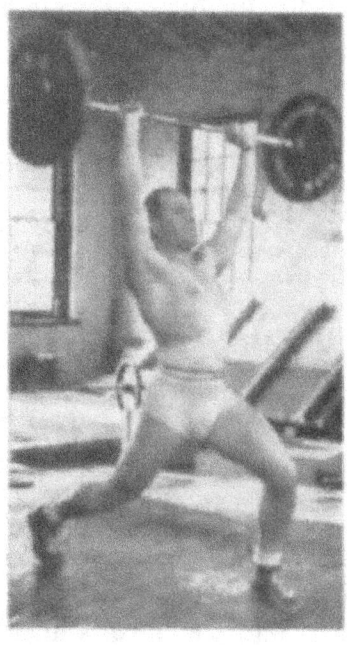

Above—Stend Olson, the greatest Danish lifter, who was breaking world's records a few years ago. At right—Good Vinablei' style in the jerk. He has clean and jerked 370 pounds.

173

TWO HANDS DEAD HANG SNATCH

LIFT NO. 35.—At the beginning of this lift, the bar is tilled to a position across the thighs with the back erect. Lowering the body, but not permitting the bell to touch the floor, the bell is brought to its proper position overhead as described in the method of performing the two hands snatch. The rules as supplied with the two hands snatch are in effect with this lift: the only variation is the starting position.

Method of Performance

The object of this lift is to develop a stronger pull, a better and higher second pull. At the start of the lift when the bell is suspended across the thighs, arms straight, back straight, the body is lowered keeping the buttocks low and the back flat. Many lifters prefer to lower the bell until it nearly touches the floor as this permits a longer pull, while others lift the weight from a position above the knees. Either position is permissible.

Causes for Disqualification Are: The same as those supplied with the rules for performing the two hands snatch.

TWO HANDS REPETITION SNATCH

LIFT No. 36.—This lift must be performed in the "dead hang" style and at least five repetitions are required. The lift must be performed as described in two hands snatching and in I he dead hang snatch.

Method of Performance This particular lift, or series of lifts, in my opinion is the best single exercise in the line of physical training. It is made a part of the fifty lifts in this book partly because it is the best means of improving two hands snatching ability, cleaning ability, and raising the standard of American weight lifting, but also because it is the best exercise known. It brings even- muscle into play, developing speed, timing, co-ordination, endurance, nerve force, balance, and sheer athletic ability. More than any other lift it builds the desirable qualities enumerated at greater length in the chapter concerning the benefits of weight lifting. The repetitions greatly increase the speed of respiration, the circulation, aid elimination and improve appetite and digestion. Any man, even if he is not interested in competitive weight lifting, will be wise to spend considerable time practicing this series of lifts for the physical benefit he will derive from it.

The object of this lift is to use the greatest poundage that practice has proven you have the best possible opportunity to succeed with for a record attempt. It is performed exactly as described for the dead hang snatch and the same causes for disqualification are in effect as for the two hands snatch.

RIGHT HAND SNATCH

LIFT No. 37.—The bar bell shall be taken from the ground to arm's length overhead in one clean movement; in " fixing " the bell the trunk may be bent to the side, and the legs to any extent, but to lock the arm by " pushing " or " pressing out " the bell shall be counted cause for disqualification. At the conclusion of the lift the trunk shall be erect, the lifting arm and the legs straight, and the feet in line not more than sixteen inches apart.

Method of Performance

As in the two hands snatch there are various methods of performing this lift. Early in my weight lifting career, with limited training, while the one hand lifts were a part of the championship program, I one hand snatched 165 when my two hands snatch record was only 150. So I believe the style that I will first offer to be the best. Stand dose to the bar with the feet about eighteen inches apart. Bend the knees slightly, bending in the back as in the two hands snatch. Prepare to grasp the bar with a slow dive and hook. The back is kept flat throughout, the hips low, as the knees are bent. Grasp the bar tightly, using the hook grip. You have concentrated on a long hard pull, determining to pull the bell as high as possible—at least to the level of the neck or chin. Start the lift with the arm straight, the initial pull being given by the back and legs. Pull with increasing rapidity, with all your force, keeping the bar close to the chest and pulling high. Immediately as the bell reaches its highest point, the body must be lowered. My style was to go into a full squat, at the same time turning a quarter turn or stepping forward a bit with the foot on the lifting side.

Close observation of lifting styles will illustrate that the final position of the bent press, the one hand snatch, and the one hand jerk arc almost identical. The knees arc well bent, the body bent over to right angles, the side upon the thigh, and the free hand either resting upon the thigh, hanging between the legs, or crossed to the opposite knee where it rests. The non-lifting hand at the beginning of the lift should be rested across the knee on its side. A sharp push is given with this non-lifting hand as the weight is lifted from the floor. It will add pounds to your record.

Some lifters will use the get set style, starting the lift after a momentary straightening and bending of the legs to give some rebound to the start of the lift. A few lifters who have succeeded with fair poundages split in one hand snatching similar to their method in two hands snatching. This method does not permit as low a position or as high a poundage as the full squat. Best to master the full squat

176

position as it will greatly assist you in performing the snatch, the jerk, the bent press and the one hand swing. To teach the body the proper position, hold the weight overhead with one hand, then lower the body into the lowest possible position—the full squat position as shown in illustration.

When the bell is fixed overhead rise immediately to the erect position. The non-lifting hand can assist in maintaining balance and helping the body to the erect position when really heavy poundages arc employed.

Causes for Disqualification Are: Pressing out or pushing as the arm is locked overhead.

The one hand snatch. Back flat, hips low, non-lifting hand on the thigh, pulling the weight high as possible, then a sudden drop to the low squat position to fix the weight overhead. Terpak lifting.

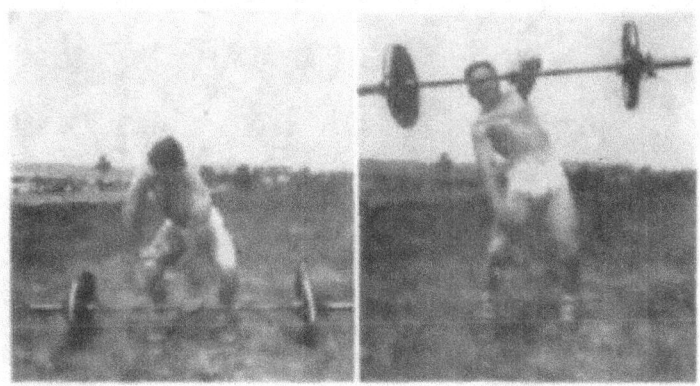

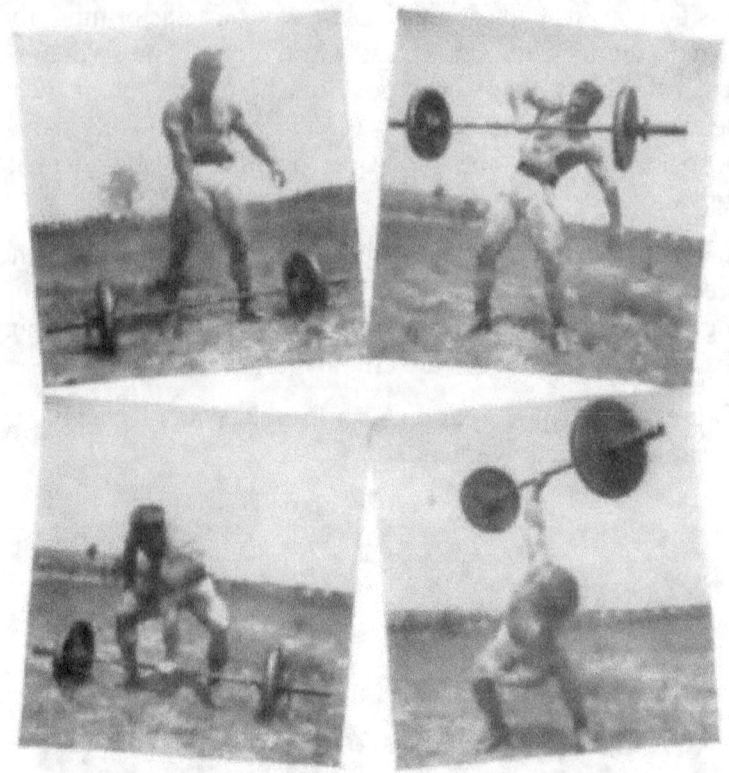

Grimek one hand snatching. About to dive for the weight, the proper starting position, pulling high, then dropping under the weight.

LEFT HAND SNATCH

LIFT NO. 38.- Details of performance identical with those offered for the right hand snatch.

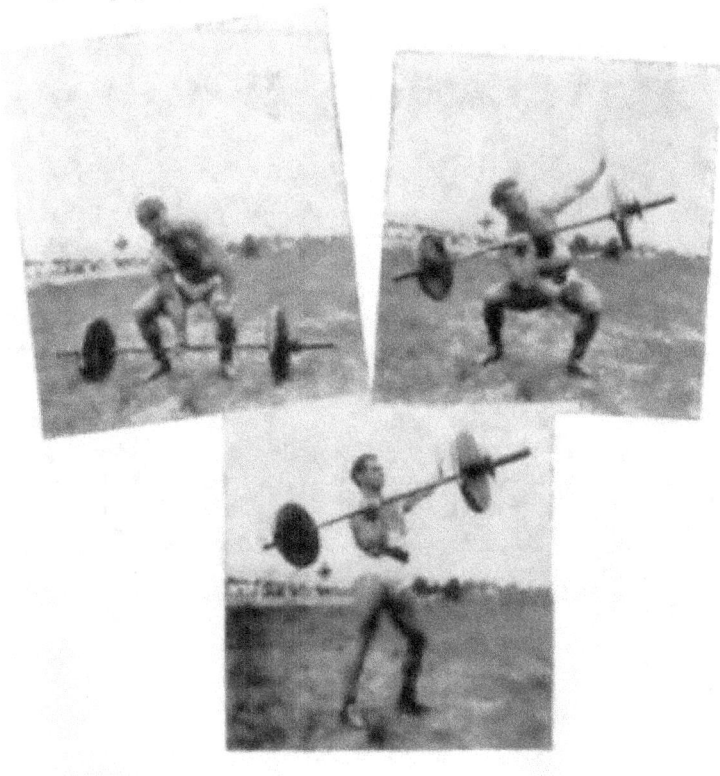

Grimek's style in the clean and jerk. The low position of his clean is especially notable.

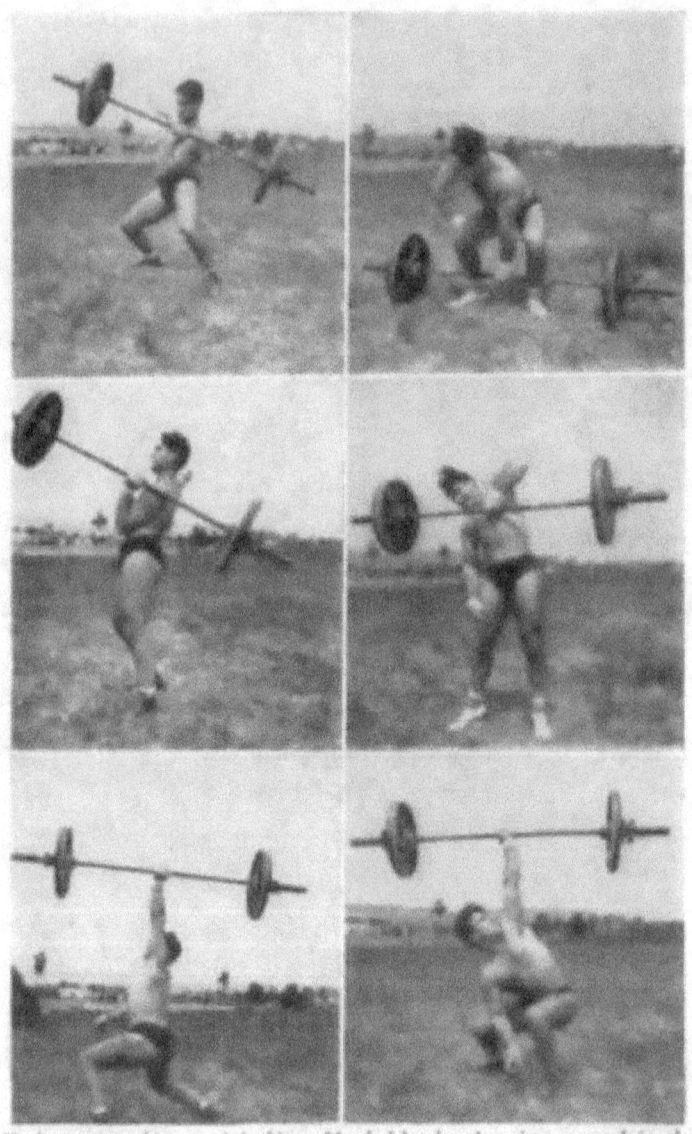

Terlazzo snatching and jerking. He holds the American record in these styles and seems capable of breaking world's records, but these lifts are no longer a part of our national championship program. In the one arm clean and jerk he is shown in the starting position, hook grip, cleaning the weight, about to jerk and getting under the weight with similar leg action to that he used in establishing his world's two hands jerk record.

LIFT No. 39.- The bar bell shall be taken to the shoulder in one clean movement and thence jerked to arm's length overhead. In the " pull in " or clean to the shoulder the trunk may be bent sideways; the elbow may rest upon the thigh, prior to standing erect, but should the bar be brought into contact with the body below the line of the nipples, it shall be counted cause for disqualification. To rest the elbow on the body prior to jerking the weight overhead is also permitted. At the conclusion of the lift the trunk shall be erect, the lifting arms and leg straight, and the heels together.

Method of Performance

Stand with the feet close to the bar about eighteen inches apart. The starting position is similar to that of the one hand snatch except that while the knuckles are front in the one hand snatch, the palm is front in the 011c hand jerk. It is best for most men to use the hook grip and the dive style. If the dive is not employed, momentarily straightening and bending of the legs will provide a certain amount of rebound. The non-lifting hand is rested upon the knee 011 its side, and gives a starting push as the weight is lifted from the floor. The legs are bent, the buttocks low, the back flat, the head fairly well up. Pull the bell hard and high so that the weight can be fixed with the elbow- on the hip if that is the style practice proves to be best for you. Heavy cleans can be made by lowering the body considerably as the weight is pulled high. The feet are turned in a quarter circle as the weight is pulled up so that it will be at right angles to the body instead of parallel with it as in the beginning. Tall men are good cleaners and seldom need be concerned with greatly lowering the body during the clean. But the shorter men in their respective bodyweight classes will find it best to squat quite low under the clean.

In jerking front the hip it is best to stand with the foot on the lifting side slightly advanced and most of the weight resting upon it. With the jerk from the hip there is usually a slight bend in the rear leg, the leg on the non-lifting side. In preparing to jerk, it is best to induce a back hang to the bell by a pressure of the hand. Turn it so that the front of the bell extends out slightly from the front of the body. The back of the bell is in the rear of the body. The bell is jerked as high as possible with a sudden sharp bending and straightening of the knees. Some lifters will split the feet as in two hands snatching, jerking or cleaning, and succeed with a good poundage.- But in jerking from the hip a better effort is possible if the body drops into the full squat position as in bent pressing and snatching.

There Is a variation of one hand jerking which is used by some, of the best performers. The elbow is not rested 011 the hip in this style, the bell against, not on. the shoulder. This permits the body to be held quite erect, the legs perfectly straight and in line as in two hands jerking. The body- being more erect, the bell much higher, it is not so difficult to jerk it to arm's length. The men who follow this method of lifting split under the weight and succeed with splendid poundages.

Causes for Disqualification Are: Bringing the bell into contact with the body below the line of the nipples, failure to hold the position in readiness to jerk the weight for two seconds.

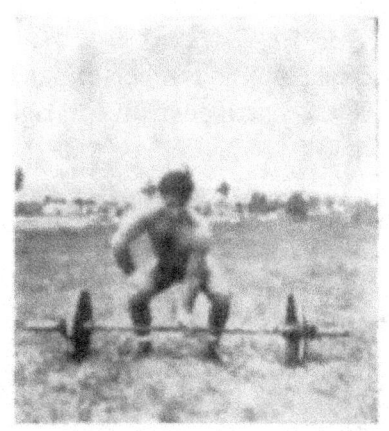

Terlazzo, at the start of the one arm clean.

Terpak one arm clean and jerking. Note the high position at which he holds the bar bell, the straightness of both legs as he prepares to jerk the weight. The bell is held high and it is not necessary to dip low in fixing the weight overhead with this style.

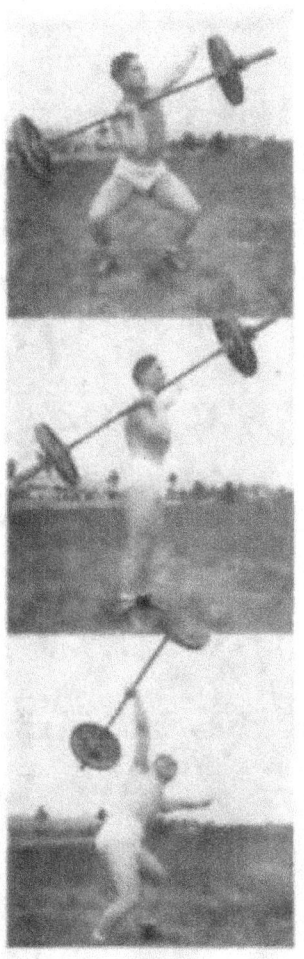

183

LIFT No. 40. Identical with the rule, method of performance and causes for disqualification as described with the right hand jerk.

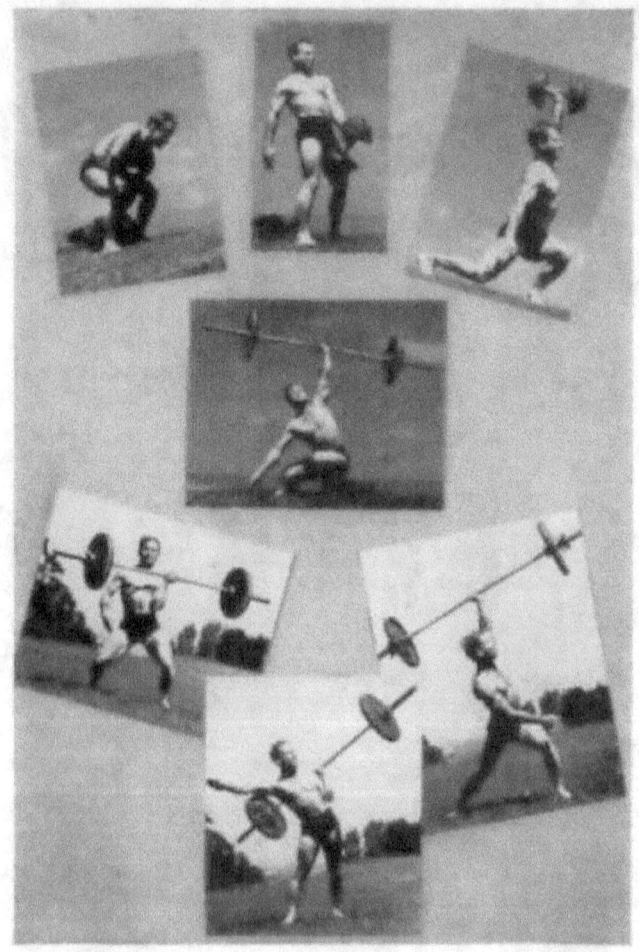

Dick Bartlett, one of the world's greatest one arm lifters, showing his form in the swing, the snatch and the clean and jerk. He snatched 22 pounds more than bodyweight, one hand jerked 55 pounds more than bodyweight.

LIFT NO. 41.—The dumbell, which at the commencement of the lift must lie at right angles to the lifter's front, shall, kept in that position throughout, be taken to arm's length overhead. The lift may be performed in one movement or a series of movements, but in the latter instance there shall be no pause between any of these movements, nor shall any part of the bell be brought into contact with the floor after it has been lifted therefrom. In "fixing" the bell the trunk and legs may be bent to any extent, and the bell may be brought into contact with the forearm; but to lock the arm by pushing shall be counted cause for disqualification.

Method of Performance

The best performers in this style of lifting load the dumbell so that the back end is loaded with as much as twenty-five pounds more than the front. When heavy-poundages are approached it is wise to use a leather gauntlet to protect the forearm and wrist. In assuming the starting position, stand with the feet about eighteen inches apart and the bell at right angles to the body. Keeping the back flat, the buttocks low, bend the knees so that the bar can be grasped with the lifting hand close to the front disk. The non-lifting hand, as in the one hand snatch and one hand clean, is placed just above the knee of the leg on its side of die body, with the fingers and thumb turned inward.

The bell is lifted until the trunk is erect, the arm remaining straight throughout, the weight equally distributed on both feet, the knees locked and the lifting shoulder raised as high as possible. When the shoulder has reached its highest position, keeping the back flat, the buttocks low, rebend the knees almost touching the floor with the lowered bell. As the body has been raised to the erect position the non-lifting hand has been held against the side of the thigh. It is now placed in its former position. When the bell has reached its lowest position, simultaneously straightening the legs and the back, pulling hard with the arm, swinging the bell upward and backward, pressing with the non-lifting hand, toss the bell to arm's length overhead. As the bell reaches the highest position to which you can pull it, split sharply forward with the leg on the lifting side. (Those lifters who habitually step forward with the left leg in cleaning, snatching and jerking, will be able to perform more creditably with the left hand than with the right.)

The heavy end of the bell will come into contact with the forearms and rest there. Some practice will be necessary to properly co-ordinate these movements. It's best to practice repetition swinging with a moderate weight first without moving the feet to accustom all the muscles to work in unison. When the bell has been fixed at arm's length, the forward foot is brought back, the feet held in line and the count taken. Some lifters will prefer to drop into the full squat position in fixing the bell overhead—a position similar to the low position in bent pressing, one hand snatching and jerking.

Causes for Disqualification Are: Failure to swing the bell clean to arm's length overhead, locking the elbow by pressing or pushing, motion not continuous where more than one movement is made, permitting the bell to touch the floor while the lift is in progress.

LEFT HAND SWING

LIFT NO. 42.—Identical with the rules and method of performance offered for the right hand swing.

TWO HANDS CLEAN AND JERK

LIFT NO. 43.—The bar bell shall be taken clean to the shoulders in one continuous movement to come to rest at the sternum bone where the collar bones meet or at any point on the chest above the nipples. The bar must not rest upon any part of the chest before coming to rest at the point from which it will be jerked. The recovery from the "pull in," preparatory for the jerk, must be speedy and continuous, and any delay in doing so shall be counted cause for disqualification. The lifter must then adopt the jerking stance with feet, if separated, held on the same plane about sixteen inches apart. In jerking the bell the extent of the lunging shall not be limited, but the recovery to the erect position must be speedy and continuous. At the conclusion of the lift the bell must be held for two seconds on locked arms overhead in the final position, motionless, with the feet on a line and not more than sixteen inches apart. The bell shall not be lowered until the referee has given the signal by clapping sharply with both hands. The recovery must be speedy and continuous, both after the clean and after the jerk. Any delay will be counted cause for disqualification.

Method of Performance

Stand with the feet close to the hell and about sixteen inches apart or closer if this seems best for you. I believe it best to stand with the knees slightly bent, the back curved well inward. Lower the body, back flat, buttocks low, head erect. Grasp the bar with hands at shoulder width apart and with a heavy poundage it's best to employ the hook grip. Concentrate on a long hard pull, pulling the bell straight up, stepping well forward when the hell reaches its highest point, thrusting the elbows well forward and fixing the bar upon the upper chest. Immediately pull back the front foot and arise to the erect position.

Stand with the feet on a line—about sixteen inches apart. Sharply bend the knees only a moderate amount; bending them too far causes the body to lean forward and will frequently result in a failure to hold the jerk. Keep the body perfectly erect, the head raised slightly; sharply straighten the legs, sending the bar as high as possible overhead. As the bell reaches its highest point overhead, split under it. Stepping well forward with the front foot, slightly back with the rear foot, push strongly throughout and hold the bar at arm's length. If the bell is jerked straight up, the front foot advanced well forward, it should he easy enough to lock the arms overhead.

Causes for Disqualification Are: Touching the bar to any part of the body below the nipples and above the knees, failure to come immediately to the erect position after the clean or the jerk, failure to stand still, holding the weight overhead for the count.

Shams, the Egyptian, attempting to jerk 325 pounds. A success with this lift would have given him the world's championship.

Kratkowski jerking 319 pounds. Bob Hoffman, who served as master of ceremonies on this occasion, is seated in the background. This was the first day on which he first pressed 250 pounds.

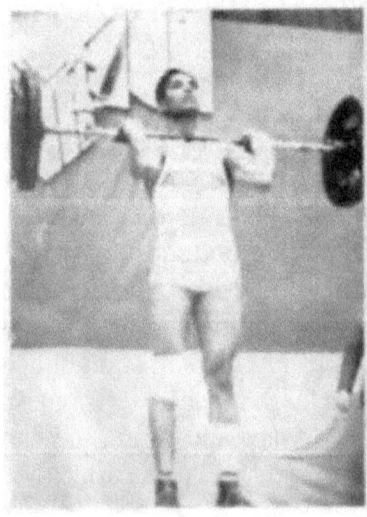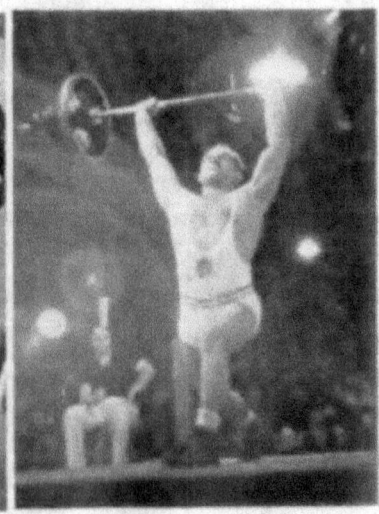

188

LIFT No. 44. The bar bell is picked up and brought to a position across the thighs, the back erect. From this position it is lowered,- not permitted to touch the floor however. and then brought back up to the clean position. The feet are brought together and held for the count. No jerk is necessary.

Method of Performance

Reach down and grasp the bell in the identical style you employ for two hands 1 leaning. Straighten up with the bar. back erect, bar resting across the thighs. Lower the bell. Some prefer to lower it until it nearly touches the floor, permitting a longer pull; others draw it from a position just above the knee. Pulling close to the body, raise it as high as possible. Lunge forward, splitting or sliding the feet fore and aft so that the bell is fixed at the shoulders as in the regular two hands clean.

Causes for Disqualification Are: 'Pouching the bell to the floor after it has been lifted from that position at the beginning of the lift, touching any part of the body between the knees and the nipples after the second stage of the lift, failing to hold the weight for the count at the completion of the lift.

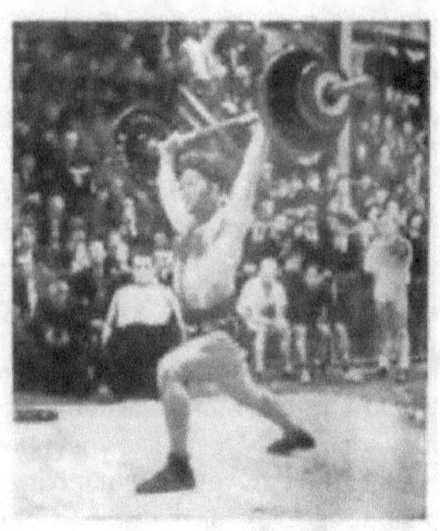

See Louie Abele starting position in the two hands clean as illustrated on page 123. Alf Hillman of the Toronto York team, Toronto, Canada, long the best middleweight lifter in the dominion, completing a heavy jerk.

TWO HANDS CONTINENTAL JERK

LIFT NO. 45.—The bar bell may be taken to the shoulders in a series of movements, and may be rested upon or against any part of the legs and trunk in so doing. A bell may also be worn to support the bell prior to turning it to the shoulders, from whence it shall be jerked to arm's length overhead. At the conclusion of the lift the trunk shall be erect, the arms and legs straight, and the heels together.

Method of Performance

Starting as in the two hands clean, with feet eighteen inches apart, standing close to the bar, Hat back, lift the bar high enough that it can be dropped behind the buckle of the belt. Stand with the feet in line, preparing to lift the weight to the chest. With a sharp bending and straightening of the legs, leaning well back with the shoulders, pull the bar high enough that the splitting of the legs front and back, lunging under the weight, will permit fixing it at the shoulders in a similar position to that assumed in the clean. Retrace the

190

front foot, feet on line and jerk the weight to arm's length as in the jerk after the clean.

The old continental lifters frequently lifted the weight to shoulders in a series of movements, actually leaning back and rolling it from waist to shoulders. But any trained lifter should be able to get more weight to the shoulders in two movements than he could possibly jerk to arm's length and hold overhead.

Causes for Disqualification Are: Failure to hold the weight at arm's length, feet in line for the count.

TWO HANDS CLEAN OR CONTINENTAL AND JERK BEHIND NECK

LIFT NO. 46.—The bar bell, having been lifted to the shoulders in either the clean or continental style, is raised overhead; then lowered behind the neck to rest upon the shoulders, shall from that position be jerked to arm's length overhead. At the conclusion of the lift the trunk shall be erect, the arms and legs straight, and heels together.

Method of Performance

Pull the weight to the upper chest in the style described in commentating or cleaning. Holding the body erect, tin- feet in line, dip sharply as in jerking the weight, stepping forward slightly, lowering the bell behind neck. In approaching a heavy poundage raise the shoulders somewhat to serve as a cushion when the bar is dropped behind neck. Take up the weight of dropping the bell by giving a bit with the body.

In jerking the weight it is optional whether you jerk front a position with the feel in line or with one of them slightly advanced. This is the only two hand lift in which it is permissible to jerk with one foot advanced. When the bell has been fixed at arm's length overhead bring the feet in line, at which position the count is taken.

Cause for Disqualification Is: Failure to hold the weight overhead for the count.

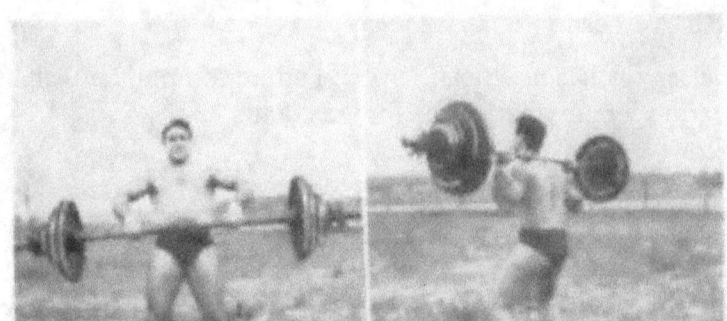

Terlazzo continenting and jerking behind neck.

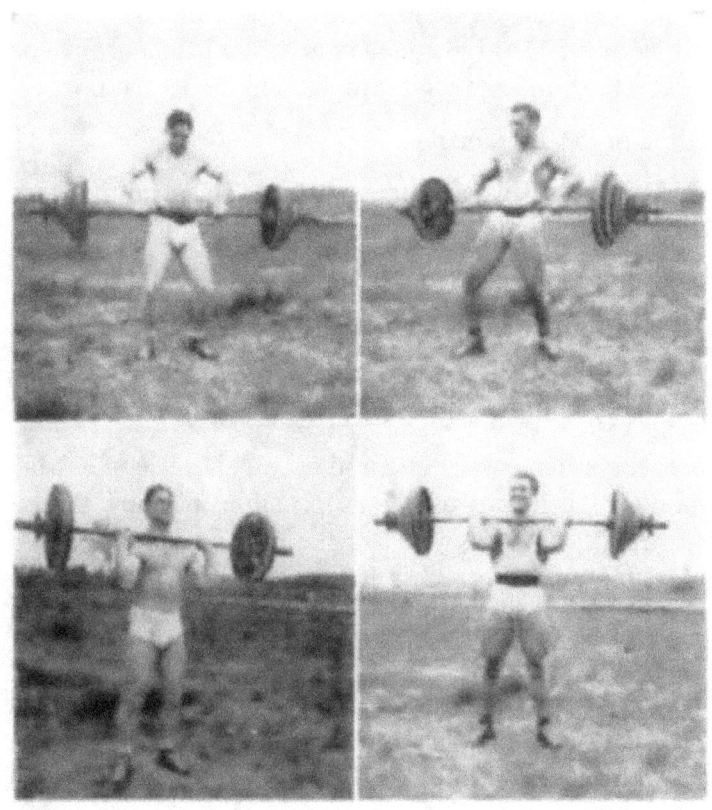

Terpak commentating and about to jerk the weight from the shoulders. His record in the jerk is 390, more than double his bodyweight. John Grimek commentating and smiling as he holds 310 pounds at his shoulder in preparation to jerk. His record in the jerk is 360 pounds.

CONTINENTAL PRESS

Lift No. 47.—The bar bell shall be taken clean to the shoulders after which the starting position shall be assumed. This position must be taken with the feet on a line about sixteen inches apart. The trunk may be inclined forward as much as desired. A pause of two seconds is made at the starting position. The bell is then pressed to arm's length overhead. /Is soon as the press begins, the legs and trunk may be bent to any extent but lowering the body vertically is not permitted. At the conclusion of the lift the trunk shall be erect, the arms and legs straight, and the feet in line.

Method of Performance

Pull the bell to the shoulders in one clean motion same style as in preparing to military press or jerk the weight. To fix the bell at the shoulder while leaning forward it is necessary that the elbows be inclined well forward. When the bell is in at the shoulders, place the feet in line, sixteen inches apart, the elbows well up, incline the body well forward and hold this position for two seconds.

When the referee has given the signal, raise the trunk, bending it backward as far as possible, pushing the bell upward ;ls strongly as you tan; the back Is bent as far bark as possible until the bell is held overhead at arm's length. When the arms are straight, raise the trunk, stand erect with the feet still on a line for the count.

Causes for Disqualification Are: Bringing the bell into contact with the body below the nipples, not holding the forward leaning, starting position for two seconds, lowering the trunk vertically while the press is being made, jerking with the legs at the start of the lift.

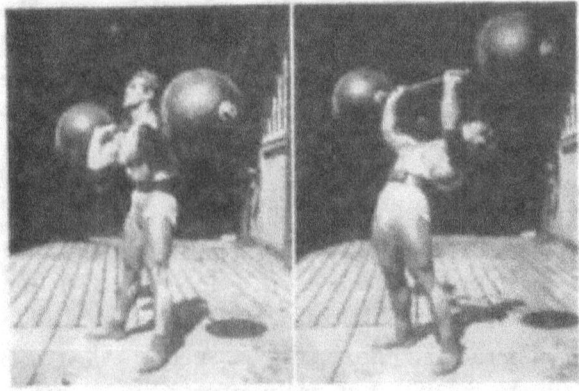

Grimek continental pressing bar bell 245.

194

LIFT NO. 48.—The barbell shall be taken to the shoulder with two hands without restriction as to method and. having been transferred into one hand, shall be grasped in the center, be elevated overhead to arm's length by means of lateral pressure. During the press from the shoulder it shall be counted cause for disqualification should any part of the bell he brought into contact with the hip. At the conclusion of the lift the trunk shall be erect, the lifting arm and legs straight, and the heels on a line about sixteen inches apart.

Method of Performance

There are a variety of ways to bring the bell to the shoulder. The majority will place the lifting hand in the center of the bell as in one hand cleaning. Place the non- lifting hand under the lifting hand thus lifting the bell to the hip or shoulder. As the majority grasp the bar at the right of the center grip, some will place the left hand on the bar close to the right hand and pull in that manner. Still others will clean the bar in the usual way, shifting the hand to the proper position to hold the bell at the shoulder. Some will prefer to rock the bar to the shoulder. This is done by standing the bar on end, having previously found the center. The thumb is rested toward the back of the neck and the bar close to the neck as possible. The non-lifting hand grasps the lower end of the bar and then the bar is pulled backward into position at the shoulder. Some will pull the bar to a position where the lifting elbow is on the front of the hip and then shift it back into position, while others pull the bell to the top of the shoulder lowering it to the pressing position behind the hip.

To assume the correct position for the bent press stand with the feet in line and the heels about sixteen inches apart a greater distance for larger men. As we are describing the right arm bent press, the right leg should be kept straight and the toe pointed straight forward. The left foot is turned outward to an angle of forty-five degrees, and the knee is bent slightly. The hip is pushed far to the side and the elbow lifted well back of it. The forearm remains perpendicular throughout the lift and the non-lifting hand in the beginning is free. Some prefer to keep the bar level, but the majority induce a considerable back hang. The bell is turned around to a point where it is parallel with the feet. This will usually place it so that it is touching the shoulder on the lifting side.

From this position the object of the lift is to fall away or bend to the left, keeping the elbow perpendicular and the upper arm on the body. This lift was originally called the " screw lift," as the body turned throughout the lift. But greater successes are made if the body is turned well around first, so that there is little more than the side and forward bend during the progress of the lift. While the majority must start and bend slowly to properly balance the bell, those who saw the immortal Arthur Saxon in action— his lift of 371 being the greatest on record—insist that he bent very quickly to the side, completing the lift as rapidly as possible.

As the body leans toward the front—the direction the left foot points—push the hip well over under the bell. The right leg remains straight until the arm is nearly straight-ened, but when the bend has reached a point where it is felt that the arm is about to leave the body the left leg is bent a bit more. When the upper arm begins to leave the body, press very strongly, keeping the bell directly over the head, turning the eyes and head so that the bell can be watched throughout. At this point the bell has a tendency to turn and your success will depend to a great extent on your ability to check its motion. It is especially difficult to press and maintain balance while the bell is turning and the body being lowered. Some lifters find it possible to check the turning of the bell by causing the bell to hang considerably from the level.

When the arm is about to lock, keep pressing as strongly as possible, bending both legs evenly, lowering the buttocks; remain in this position until the bell is very definitely balanced overhead. To reach the extreme low position it is best to twist the body so that the shoulder goes down between the legs. Some lifters can keep the non-lifting hand I on the left knee, but the majority can not get low enough in this position. The shoulder passes down below the knee on the non-lifting side, the hand remaining either in suspension or extended across to rest on the right knee.

In my early years of bent pressing, when I first passed two hundred pounds, 1 found it necessary to slide the hand down the thigh and knee, then to rest upon the knee with the side of my upper body, finally to raise up a bit, get my hand under me and thus steady myself and push up.

Every man is not best suited for bent pressing, but any man can become a good performer in this style. I do not believe that I am exactly suited for it. The comparatively short upper arm which makes me a poor military presser (I'm the only man in the world who jerked to arm's length double what I could press) also prevents me from putting my elbow on the hip in the proper pressing position. It is especially difficult for me to prevent the bar from turning owing to my position; yet I succeeded with an official lift after my fortieth birthday of 263 pounds, which is a modern world's record at present.

While arising with the weight keep the eyes on the bell, bring the feet in line and hold the weight for the count.

In lowering the weight, shift the grip so that both hands grasp the bar in the position used in two hands jerking.

Lower the bar to chest and from there to the floor. This lift is one which is interesting to contestant and spectator alike. It will give you a real reputation as a strong man. Most any man can learn to press more in this style with one hand than in the military style with two. I11 fact some men have succeeded in bent pressing more than they could clean and jerk. At present this lift is much in favor. It builds great bodily strength, teaches balance to a superlative degree and must be considered one of the key lifts as the body is in the lowest possible position in lifting.

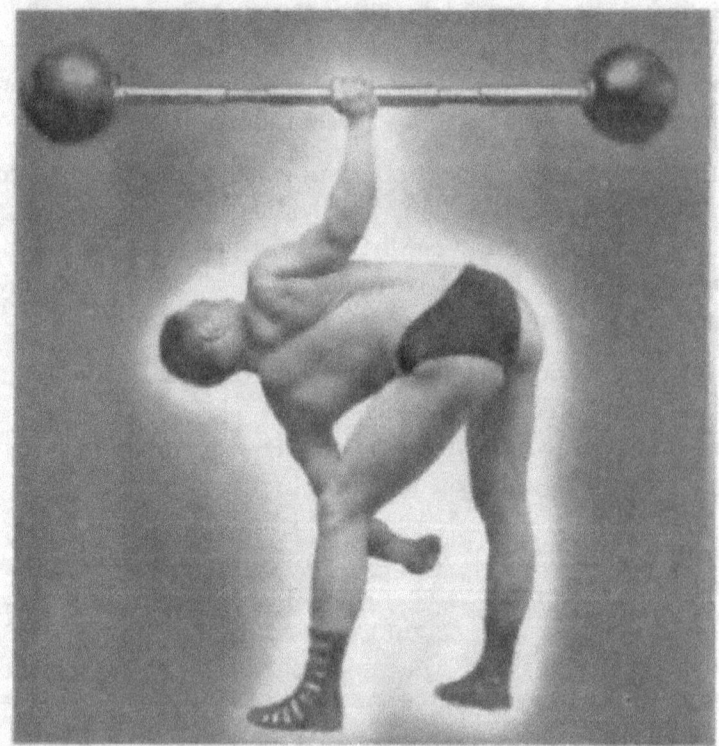

Bob Harley, of Siegmund Klein's gym, the winner of the New York City bent press contest who, in the opinion of the author, has the best style in the bent press. His record is 230 pounds.

TWO HANDS TO SHOULDER AND LEFT ARM BENT PRESS

LIFT NO. 49.—Exactly the same as with the right hand bent press except that the opposite arm is used in pressing.

TWO HANDS ANYHOW

LIFT No. 50.—The bar bell and ring weight or dumbell shall be lifted to arm's length overhead " anyhow." For example, the bar bell may be taken to the shoulder with two hands, thence to be jerked or bent pressed overhead, after which the kettle bell, ring weight or dumbell is lifted to arm's length. Again, the bar bell may be taken to arm's length overhead with two arms, then transferred into one hand, after which the ring weight, kettle bell or dumbell is taken to arm's length with the other hand. At the conclusion of the lift the trunk shall be erect, both arms straight and parallel with each other, the legs straight and the heels on a line.

Method of Performance

From the rule you can see that several methods are employed in getting the bar bell to single arm length overhead, but the most common style will be described at greatest length. Clean and jerk the bar bell to arm's length as described in the performance of that lift. Stand with the feet astride and the kettle bell about six inches in front of the line of the toes. When you have the kettle bell in the proper position, transfer your attention to the bell you are holding at arm's length. Bending the left knee slightly, shift the weight of the bell over that leg; maintain the right leg straight. The bell will be in a slanting position when it is shifted to the left of the center of the bell. When the weight is well placed over the left leg, straighten tha" knee. Holding the left arm straight prepare to shift the grip of the right hand, bend the right leg to assist in gripping the bar in the new position, then straighten the right leg, placing the weight again over the left leg. If the grip has not been shifted properly the bell will have a back bang. Push up the hang with the disengaged hand, gradually shifting the weight to the proper balance. When the bell has been properly fixed, well balanced, bend down and slowly reach for the kettle bell. Leaning so that the weight is over the left foot press the kettle bell to arm's length. Here the count of two is taken. You will find it easier to complete the final stages of the lift if a front hang of the bar is continued, although this is not essential.

Should the bent press style be used with the anyhow style (this is the method used by Arthur Saxon in lifting the greatest weight ever hoisted to arm's length by man— 336-pound bar bell, 112-pound kettle bell,—448 in all) lift the bell to the shoulder in the two hands style. Press it to arm's length, and then when it is properly balanced reach down and get the kettle bell. Raise to the erect position, pressing it to arm's length and holding it for the count.

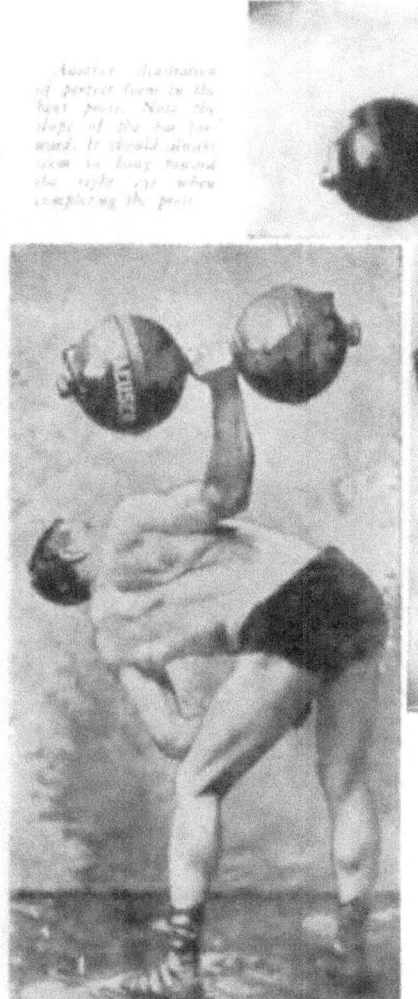